Biomaterials in Surgery

Biomaterials in Surgery

Edited by
G. H. I. M. Walenkamp

With Contributions by

F. C. Bakker
D. J. Bakker
C. A. van Blitterswijk
S. J. M. Bouwmeester
J. D. de Bruijn
S. K. Bulstra
H. Büchner
Å. S. Carlsson
B. Chevallay
W. Ege
A. Göpferich
R. Göttmann
U. Grüßner
H. J. Th. M. Haarman
D. Herbage
N. H. M. Hoefnagels
Ch. Jürgens
S. Kaarsemaker
I. Kreiser-Saunders
H.-R. Kricheldorf

R. Kuijer
K.-D. Kühn
S. Lösel
H. Maurer
A. Moser
R. van den Munckhof
B. Nies
H.-J. Pfefferle
St. Roche
J. Schmidt
H. G. K. Schmidt
E. C. Shors
C. H. Siebert
C. Tuchscherer
M. Vert
G. H. I. M. Walen-
  kamp
R. Wenz
R. J. Wolvius

76 figures in 147 single illustrations
31 tables

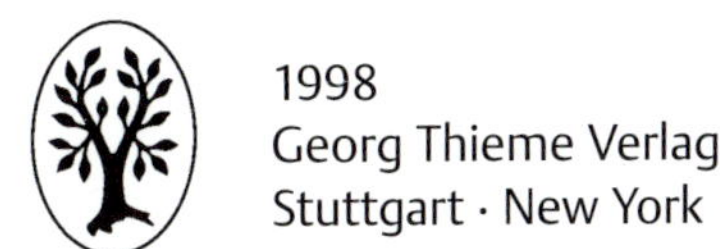

1998
Georg Thieme Verlag
Stuttgart · New York

Die Deutsche Bibliothek –
CIP-Einheitsaufnahme

Biomaterials in Surgery : 31 tables / ed. by
G. H. I. M. Walenkamp. With contributions
by F. C. Bakker … – Stuttgart ; New York :
Thieme, 1998

1998 Georg Thieme Verlag
Rüdigerstraße 14
D-70469 Stuttgart

Printed in Germany

Typesetting: DataSatz Roßberg, Metzingen
  System: 3B2 (4.62)
Cover Design: Martina Berge, Erbach-Ernsbach
Graphics: Barbara Gay, Stuttgart
Printing: Grammlich, Pliezhausen
Bookbinding: F. W. Held, Rottenburg

ISBN 3-13-104791-7

1 2 3 4 5 6

Adresses

Dr. C. A. van Blitterswijk
Leiden University
Biomaterials Research Group
Prof. Bronkhorstlaan 10, Bld. 57
3723 MB Bilthoven
The Netherlands

Dr. J. D. de Bruijn
Leiden University
Biomaterials Research Group
Prof. Bronkhorstlaan 10, Bld. 57
3723 MB Bilthoven
The Netherlands

Dr. S. K. Bulstra
Department of Orthopaedic Surgery
University Hospital Maastricht
PO Box 5800
6202 AZ Maastricht
The Netherlands

Å. S. Carlsson, MD
Department of Orthopaedic Surgery
Malmö University Hospital
20502 Malmö
Sweden

Dr. W. Ege
Wissenschaftlicher Berater
Heraeus Kulzer GmbH
Mailänder Straße 18
60598 Frankfurt
Germany

Prof. Dr. A. Göpferich
Lehrstuhl für Pharmazeutische Technologie
Naturwissenschaftliche Fakultät IV
Chemie und Pharmazie
93040 Regensburg
Germany

Dr. U. Grüßner
Merck Biomaterial GmbH
Frankfurter Straße 250
64271 Darmstadt
Germany

Dr. D. Herbage
Centre National de la Recherche Scientifique
Institut de Biologie et Chimie des Protéines
7, passage du Vercors
69367 Lyon Cedex 07
France

Priv.-Doz. Dr. Ch. Jürgens
Abteilung für Unfall- und
Wiederherstellungschirurgie
Krankenhaus Itzehoe
Robert-Koch-Straße 2
25524 Itzehoe
Germany

Dr. A. Moser
Chirurgische Klinik
St. Josef-Hospital
Gudrunstraße 56
44791 Bochum
Germany

Dr. B. Nies
Merck Biomaterial GmbH
Frankfurter Straße 250
64271 Darmstadt
Germany

P. Patka, MD
Department of Surgery
University Hospital VU
De Boelelaan 1117
1007 MB Amsterdam
The Netherlands

H.-J. Pfefferle
Merck Biomaterial GmbH
Frankfurter Straße 250
64271 Darmstadt
Germany

Dr. H. G. K. Schmidt
Abteilung für Unfall- und
Wiederherstellungschirurgie
BG-Unfallkrankenhaus
Bergedorfer Straße 10
21033 Hamburg
Germany

Priv.-Doz. Dr. J. Schmidt
Klinik und Poliklinik für Orthopädie
Universität zu Köln
Joseph-Stelzmann-Straße 9
50924 Köln
Germany

E. C. Shors, PhD
Interpore International
181 Technology Drive
Irvine California, 92 718 – 2402
USA

Dr. M. Vert
Centre de Recherche Surfactant les Biopolymères
Artificiels, URA CNRS 1465 Faculté de Pharmacie
Université de Montpellier I
15, Avenue Charles-Flahault
34060 Montpellier Cedex 1
France

G. H. I. M. Walenkamp, MD, PhD
Department of Orthopaedic Surgery
University Hospital Maastricht
P. O. Box 5800
6202 AZ Maastricht
The Netherlands

Dr. R. Wenz
Merck Biomaterial GmbH
Frankfurter Straße 250
64271 Darmstadt
Germany

Preface

There is today an increasing interest in biomaterials in most surgical disciplines. However, foreign materials have been used in the body since the beginning of this century: glass, bakelite, rubber, and many metals have been used, especially in joint reconstruction. Since then, increasing applications have shown that not only are mechanical aspects decisive for success, but especially the biological properties of the material. From the beginning differences between **bio-incompatible** and **bio-tolerant** materials became clear. Some materials, such as titanium, appeared to be **bio-inert:** there was no fibrous encapsulation of the material by the body. With these kinds of biomaterials, mainly metals and plastics, extensive experience was gained in the 70's and 80's, especially in joint replacements: hip prostheses and bone cement. About 10 years ago, new biomaterials were developed and clinical applications explored for **bio-active** and **biodegradable** materials. The applications of, e.g., growth factors in these materials are now largely tested. Fascinating developments are an illustration of a more biological approach in biomaterial use of today, and exciting new fields in patient care are being explored now. Application in orthopedic and traumatic surgery requires a thorough, scientifically-based knowledge of the physical, biochemical, as well as the biological properties of the material.

The contributions in this book were presented at a congress held in Maastricht in October 1996. We thought that it could be valuable to publish these presentations in this book form, building a bridge between recent experimental results with biomaterials and the possibilities and needs of the clinical field in the near future.

First, results are presented with well-known biomaterials such as **bone cement** and **collagen,** especially the possibility to release different drugs, and the results in total hip replacement. Secondly, new developments in applications of **ceramics** and **resorbable polymers** are presented. A growing number of these materials are available, with confusing differences in properties. Basic research indicates some interesting possibilities, especially as bone substitutes.

Hence, this book will offer the interested reader several aspects of biomaterials, as used in orthopedic and traumatic surgery, in the recent past and in the near future. Basic as well as clinical aspects are presented.

February 1998   G. H. I. M. Walenkamp

Contents

The Biomaterial Collagen

Collagen-Based Biomaterials and Tissue Engineering

B. Chevallay, St. Roche, D. Herbage

Introduction

The extracellular matrix of connective tissues is composed of molecules belonging to four families of proteins: collagens, proteoglycans, glycoproteins, and elastin. Collagen, the single most abundant protein in mammals, accounting for about 30% of all proteins, provides the principal source of mechanical strength in tissues such as bone, cartilage, skin, tendon, and ligament and contributes a structural framework to other tissues such as blood vessels and most organs (For reviews, see Burgeson and Nimni, 1992; van der Rest et al., 1993; Prockop and Kivirikko, 1995; Brown and Timpl, 1995). The generally accepted definition of a collagen is that it is a structural protein of the extracellular matrix which contains one or more domains having the conformation of a triple helix. The collagen triple helix has a coiled-coil structure made of three parallel chains with a left-handed helix assembled around a central axis and forming a right-handed super helix. The primary structure of a collagen triple helix can be written as (Gly-X-Y), since for steric reasons only glycine can occupy a position in the center of the helix. The presence of other amino acids in the Gly position alters the stability or the conformation of the helix and has been shown to be responsible for genetic diseases such as osteogenesis imperfecta (type I collagen) or chondrodysplasias (type II collagen).

In human tissues 19 different types of collagen have been identified so far corresponding to at least 33 separate genes (Table **1**). The collagen molecules can be assembled in homotrimers or heterotrimers and form multimolecular aggregates. The best known subfamily of collagens forms quarter-staggered fibrils (collagen types I, II, III, V, and XI). It is well established that these fibrillar collagens have primarily a structural, mechanical function in extracellular matrices, but recent results have shown that cell behavior (such as attachment, spreading, migration, growth, differentiation, and metabolic activity) is regulated not only by circulating molecules (hormones, growth factors, or cytokines) but also by interactions with extracellular matrix molecules including the collagens. Specific receptors on cell surfaces, such as integrins, direct the cell-matrix interactions (Juliano and Haskill, 1993; Tuckwell and Humphries, 1993; Gumbiner, 1996). Certain extracellular matrix constituents such as collagens interact with integrins in a conformation-dependent manner in which both the linear structure and spatial arrangement of the polypeptides are important for the formation of active binding sites (Kühn and Eble, 1994). Furthermore, the integrin cytoplasmic domain interacts with the cytoskeleton and is involved in signal transduction processes. These impressive advances in our understanding of cell-matrix interactions or cell behavior provide us with improved explanations of the biological activities of collagen-based biomaterials and open the way to possible developments of new biomaterials more adapted to specific functions in tissue engineering for the creation of new biological substitutes that restore, maintain, or improve tissue function (Langer and Vacanti, 1993).

Collagen as Biomaterial

Collagen is one of the oldest natural polymers that has been used by humans. World production of bovine hides and skins in 1990 amounted to nearly 4.7 million metric tons. Raw hides and skins, and bones are used commercially to produce leather, fur goods, and gelatin. The quantity of collagen used in this way amounts to over 1.5 million tons dry material and lies close to the volume of the processing of wool. Soluble gelatin is prepared by denaturation and partial degradation of the collagen present in bone and hide by acid and alkaline processing. Gelatin finds applications in the photographic, food, and pharmaceutical industries.

Table **1** The collagen types

Structure formed	Type number	Gene	Chromosome	Molecular formulas	Expression
Quarter-staggered fibrils	Type I	Col 1 A1	17q21.3-q22	$[\alpha_1\,(I)]_3$	Dentin, skin (minor form)
		Col 1 A2	7q21.3-q22	$[\alpha_1(I)]_2\alpha_2(I)$	Most connective tissues
	Type II	Col 2 A1	12q13-q14	$[\alpha_1(II)]_3$	Cartilage, vitreous humor
	Type III	Col 3 A1	2q24.3-q31	$[\alpha_1(III)]_3$	Soft connective tissues, e.g. skin, lung, vascular tissues
	Type V/XI	Col 5 A1	9q34.2-q34.3	$[\alpha_1(V)]_3$	Chinese hamster lung cells
		Col 5 A2	2q24.3-q31	$[\alpha_1(V)]_2\alpha_2(V)$	Most type I collagen containing tissues
		Col 5 A3		$\alpha_1(V)\alpha_2(V)\alpha_3(V)$	Placenta
		Col 11 A1	1 p21	$\alpha_1(XI)\alpha_2(XI)\alpha_3(XI)$	Tissues containing type II collagen
		Col 11 A2	6 p21.2	$[\alpha_3(XI) = \alpha_1(II)]$	
Basement membrane network	Type IV	Col 4 A1	13q34	$[\alpha_3(IV)]_3$	Basement membranes
		Col 4 A2	13q34	$[\alpha_1(IV)]_2\alpha_2(IV)$	
		Col 4 A3	2q35-q37	$[\alpha_3(IV)]_3$	
		Col 4 A4	2q35-q37	$[\alpha_3(IV)]_2\alpha_4(IV)$	
		Col 4 A5	Xq22		
		Col 4 A6	Xq22		
Hexagonal lattices	Type VIII	Col 8 A1	3q12-q13.1	$[\alpha_1(VIII)]_2\alpha_2(VIII)]$	Descemet's membrane endothelial cells
		Col 8 A2	1 p32.3-p34.3		
	Type X	Col 10 A1	6q21-q22	$[\alpha_1(X)_3]$	Hypertrophic cartilage
Beaded filaments	Type VI	Col 6 A1	21q22.3	$\alpha_1(VI)\alpha_2(VI)\alpha_3(VI)$	Most connective tissues
		Col 6 A2	21q22.3		
		Col 6 A3	2q37		
Fibril associated (FACIT)	Type IX	Col 9 A1	6q12-q13	$\alpha_1(IX)\alpha_2(IX)\alpha_3(IX)$	Cartilage, vitreous humor
		Col 9 A2	1 p32		
		Col 9 A3	20q13.3		
	Type XII	Xol 12 A1	6	$[\alpha_1(XII)]_3$	Tissues containing type I collagen
	Type XIV	Col 14 A1		$[\alpha_1(XIV)]_3$	
Anchoring fibrils	Type VII	Col 7 A1	3 p21	$[\alpha_1(VII)]_3$	Mesenchyme – epithelium junctions
Cell-bound ?	Type XVII	Col 17 A1	10q24.3		Skin hemidesmosomes
	Type XIII	Col 13 A1	10q22	?	Many tissues
	Type XV	Col 15 A1	9q21-q22		Many tissues
	Type XVI	Col 16 A1	1 p34-p35		Many tissues
	Type XVIII	Col 18 A1	21q22.3		Liver, kidney, placenta
	Type XIX	Col 19 A1	6q12-q14		Rhabdomyosarcoma cells

Two types of collagen-based biomaterials can be considered: (a) biomaterials retaining the native tissular structure and used as sutures, heart valves, vascular and ligament prostheses, or abdominal patches, and (b) biomaterials prepared from purified collagen, associated or not with other macromolecular components and reconstituted under different physical forms (Table **2**) (see reviews by Sabelman, 1985; Werkmeister and Ramshaw, 1992; Miyata et al., 1992). The most important source of collagen is the skin or tendon of young animals such as calf, pig, horse, or sheep. Collagen type I, the most abundant form, is extracted from dermis by treatment with an acidic solution or after a mild pepsin treatment to remove the N- and C-terminal telopeptides and then purified by sequential precipitation with salt solutions at neutral and acid pH values.

The main advantages of the use of collagen as a biomaterial are based on its role in cell-matrix interaction, its high biocompatibility and low immunogenicity, and the easy control of its biodegradability using cross-linking agents (chemical

Composition	Form	Applications
Collagen	Solution gel	Cosmetic use
		Injectable in skin cosmetic defects
		Drug delivery
		Vitreous replacement
		Viscosurgery
		Coating of bioprostheses
		3 D cell culture
	Sponge	3 D cell culture
		Wound dressing
		Hemostatic agent
		Dermal equivalent
		Drug delivery
	Hoallow fiber	Cell culture matrix
	Tubing	Tubular tissues substitutes
		Nerve regeneration
	Microsphere	Microcarrier for cell culture
	Sphere	Drug delivery system
	Membrane	Wound dressing
		Tissue guided regeneration
		Dialysis membrane
		Patches
		Corneal shield
		Spinal surgery
		Anti adhesion
	Rigid foam	Bone repair
Collagen + glycosaminoglycans	Sponges	3 D cell culture
		Wound dressing
		Dermal equivalent
	Membrane	Tissue guided regeneration
		Patches
Collagen + hydroxyapatite	Powder	Bone filling and repair
	Sponge	Drug delivery system (BMP)

Table **2**   Collagen-based biomaterials and their applications

and/or physical). Glutaraldehyde is now the most widely-used reagent but its potential cytotoxicity and induction of calcification led to the evaluation of other cross-linking agents (Table **3**). We compared the cross-linking efficiency of glutaraldehyde (GTA) hexamethylene diisocyanate (HMDC), two carbodiimides [cyanamide and 1-ethyl-3-(3-dimethylaminopropyl)-carbodiimide (EDC)], and the two acyl azide methods, developed in our laboratory (Petite et al., 1990; 1994), on type I collagen molecules in the form of gels, sponges, and films (Rault et al., 1996). The level of cross-linking was evaluated by both measuring the thermal stability by differential scanning calorimetry (DSC) and the susceptibility to collagenase degradation of the final material. As shown on Table **4** it was demonstrated that cross-linked collagen sponges and films can be prepared by the different agents in the following

order: cyanamide < EDC < hydrazine < HMDC = DPPA < GTA.

Olde Damink (1993) has shown that addition of N-hydroxysuccinimide to an EDC-containing cross-linking solution resulted in a dermal sheep collagen with a very high increase in thermal stability. Furthermore, our results with an organotypic culture model (Petite et al., 1995) and those of van Wachem et al. (1994) with a methyl cellulose cell culture system and after subcutaneous implantation in rats, demonstrate that collagen biomaterials treated with acyl azide or carbodiimide (EDC) have a better biocompatibility than the same biomaterials treated with GTA or diisocyanate. Cross-linking with polyepoxy compounds gave collagen biomaterials with interesting physical and biological properties (Miyata et al., 1992).

Table **3**   Cross-linking of collagen

Physical treatment
UV irradiation (254 nm)
γ-ray irradiation
Dehydrothermal treatment

Chemical treatment	Reagent
Bifunctional agent	
aldehyde	ex: glutaraldehyde (GTA)
diisocyanate	ex: hexamethylene diisocyanate (HMDC)
polyepoxy	ex: polyglycerol polyglycidyl ether
Activation of carboxylic acid groups	
carbodiimide	ex: cyanamide 1-ethyl-3-(3-dimethylaminopropyl)- carbodiimide HCl (EDC)
acyl azide method	ex: hydrazine diphenylphosphoryl azide (DPPA)

Table **4**   Thermal transition temperature and resistance to collagenase of collagen sponges and films non-cross-linked or cross-linked with different agents

Conditions of maximum reticulation				Thermal transition temperature (maximum)	Resistance to collagenase (30 min digestion time)
Reticulation agent	Concentration %, w/v	pH	Duration (h)	Peak (°C)	Digestion %
Sponge					
none	–	–	–	48.9 ± 0.2	80
cyanamide	1	6.2	24	60.5 ± 0.6	75
EDC	1	5.5	24	$61 \ \pm 0.5$	50
HMDC	1	5.5	96	70.8 ± 5.3	45
GTA	1	6.2	24	75.3 ± 0.6	5
Hydrazine	1	–	24	64.3 ± 4.0	55
DPPA	0.5	DMF	24	69.2 ± 2.5	55
Film					
none	–	–	–	$52 \ \pm 1.7$	85
cyanamide	1	6.2	24	58.5 ± 5.2	70
GTA	0.6	6.2	96	74.6 ± 1.5	6
hydrazine	1	–	24	69.9 ± 0.6	8
DPPA	0.5	DMF	24	72.6 ± 1.0	8

Collagen-Based Matrices in Tissue Engineering

One approach in tissue engineering for the replacement or total regeneration of damaged or missing tissues is the creation of open systems with (essentially autologous) cells placed on or within matrices. The matrices are prepared from natural materials such as collagen or from synthetic polymers and are implanted and become incorporated in the body (Langer and Vacanti, 1993).

The preparation of recombinant growth and differentiation factors (BMP, PDGF, TGF-β, etc.) allows the design of an optimal combination of signals to initiate and promote development of specialized tissues such as bone, cartilage, or skin. Indeed, the three principal ingredients for successful tissue engineering are regulatory signals, cells, and the extracellular matrix as postulated by Reddi (1994).

In this last section, we will summarize recent approaches using this concept for the regeneration of skin and cartilage and for the formation of neo-organs or organoids of potential use in gene therapy.

Skin Equivalent

In the presence of dermis, the epidermis destroyed as, for example, in a first-degree burn, regenerates spontaneously within several days. Full-thickness skin loss results in wound contraction and scar formation. Several burn centers use the method of Green et al. (1979) for the growth of human epidermal cells into multiple epithelia suitable for grafting. A normal epidermis was reformed after transplantation. However, although some sort of neo-dermis beneath the cultured epidermis was observed, the resulting cover is fragile and the lack of functional underlying dermis creates severe scarring (Heimbach et al., 1988). For these reasons several authors have proposed skin substitutes made of collagen-based matrices seeded or not with fibroblasts and combined or not with autologous epidermal cells (see reviews by Yannas, 190; Prunieras, 1991; Bell, 1995). For example Bell et al. (1981) proposed the culture of fibroblasts in a collagen gel. A tissue-like matrix was formed *in vitro* by contraction of the gel. Use of human collagen has been reported (Auger et al., 1995). A different approach, followed by different authors, is the preparation of collagen-based membranes or sponges as an artificial dermis. A complex of collagen and chondroitin 6-sulfate with a silicone membrane was first reported by Yannas and Burke (1980). Several modifications of this technique have been described by other groups using collagen-GAG (Boyce et al., 1988; Suzuki et al., 1990), collagen-elastin (de Vries et al., 1995), collagen-gelatin (Koide et al., 1993), collagen-GAG-fibronectin (Doillon et al., 1987), or collagen-GAG-chitosan (Shahabeddin et al., 1990). These dermal equivalents, transformed into skin models after seeding with keratinocytes, have been proposed for pharmacological and toxicological studies or for human wound coverage.

Cartilage Repair

Pure chondral defects have a poor potential for intrinsic repair with little cellular infiltration. In contrast, an osteochondral defect results from the formation of a fibrocartilage different from hyaline cartilage in composition and structural organization and unable to restore the biomecha-

nical properties of normal articular cartilage. Recently, deep cartilage defects in the knee of young patients (under age 50) have been successfully treated with autologous chondrocyte transplantation (Brittberg et al., 1994). Healthy chondrocytes obtained from an uninvolved area of the injured knee during arthroscopy were expanded for 2 – 3 weeks *in vitro* before injection in the defect and covering with a sutured periosteal flap. Successful results were obtained in 84% of the patients with a mean follow-up of 60 months. However, it is not yet known if this method is applicable to older subjects with degenerative joint disease (osteoarthritis). Therefore, a new approach to cartilage repair proposed transplanting chondrocytes seeded within biocompatible 3 D matrices. Several groups (Freed et al., 1993; Chu et al., 1995; Sittinger et al., 1996) chose synthetic polymers such as polylactic acid (PLA) or polyglycolic acid (PGA). Our group and others (Nixon et al., 1993; Toolan et al., 1996; Fujisato et al., 1996) utilized porous collagen matrices seeded with chondrocytes as an implant for cartilage repair. Our first results (Roche et al., unpublished results) demonstrate the growth of human chondrocytes (patients over age 60) within collagen sponges cross-linked by the acyl azide method (DPPA) with a 3 – 5 fold increase in cell number after 4 weeks and a minimal dedifferentiation in the presence of ascorbate.

An another possible technique for human chondrocyte proliferation and cartilage phenotype expression was described by Frondoza et al. (1996); it involves a collagen microcarrier suspension culture system. Long-term clinical trials are needed to determine the potential of these biomaterials.

Formation of Organoids or Neo-Organs for *in vivo* Protein Delivery

In order to introduce mammalian cells as carriers of modified genetic information into hosts, Thomson et al. (1989) described the formation of organoid neovascular structures using polytetrafluoroethylene fibers coated with collagen and heparin binding growth factor 1 implanted in the peritoneal cavity of the rat. Moullier et al. (1993) developed the technique and obtained correction of lysosomal storage in the liver and spleen of MPS VII mice by implantation of skin fibroblasts engineered for human β-glucuronidase synthesis. This procedure created long-term autologous implants of genetically-modified fibro-

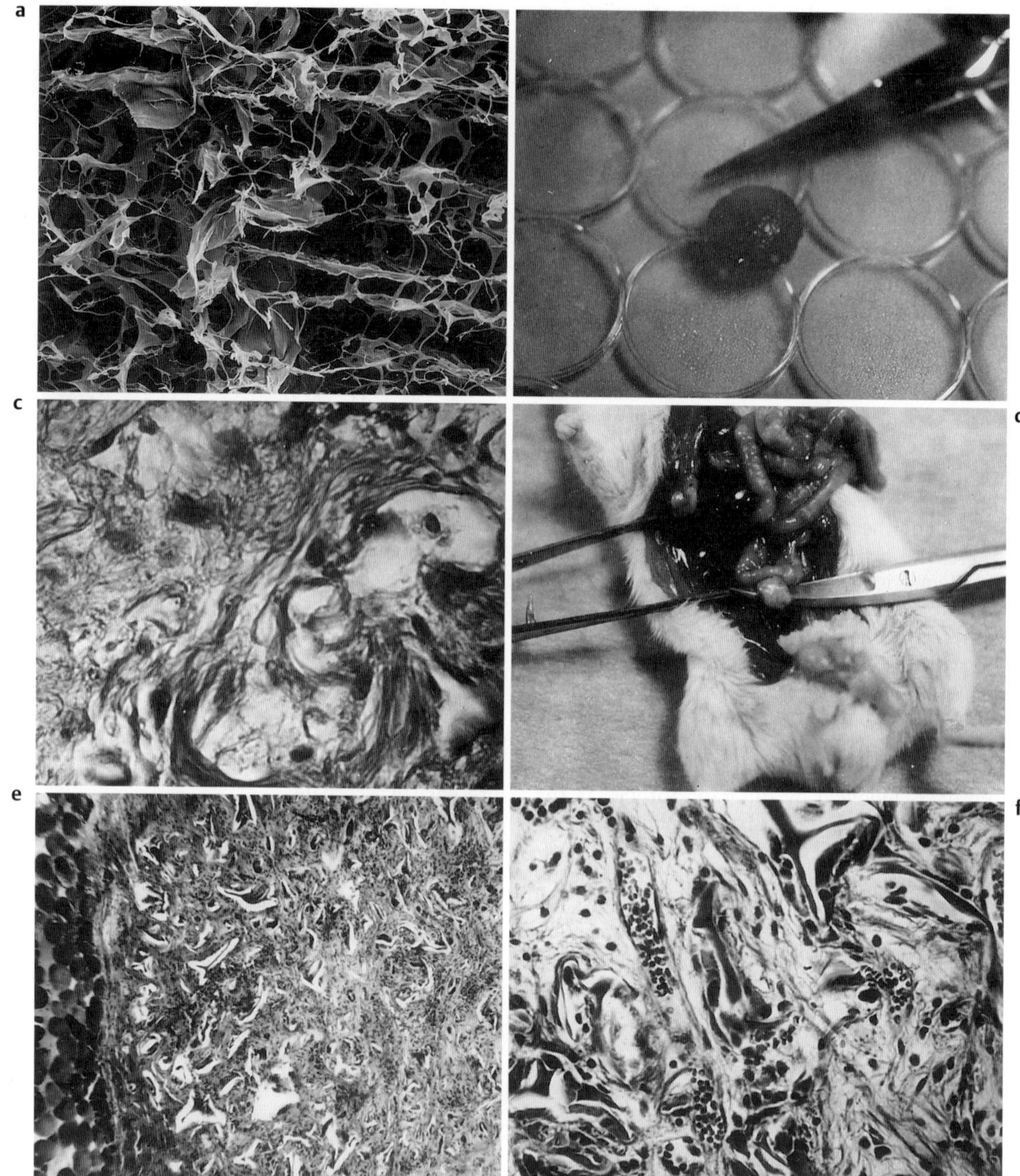

Fig. 1 (a) Collagen sponge structure (SEM) × 100. (b) Collagen sponge seeded with fibroblasts and (c) incubated 20 days *in vitro* × 650. (d) Collagen sponge with fibroblasts after 3 months intraperitoneal implantation in mouse. (e, f) Histological analysis of the sponge showing (e) attachment to the peritoneum (on the left) × 200 and (f) internal vascularization × 550.

blasts and was adapted for long-term delivery of lysosomal enzyme or erythropoietin in mice or dogs and was proposed for the treatment of Hurler's disease in patients deficient in α-L-iduronidase (Moullier et al., 1995). In our laboratory (Chevallay et al., unpublished results) we observed that collagen sponges, seeded with syngeneic fibroblasts, attached to the peritoneal cavity in mice and formed vascularized neo-organs, even in the absence of coating with heparin and/or basic fibroblast growth factor (Fig. **1**). Furthermore, cross-linked collagen sponges present a long-term stability and unmodified mechanical resistance allowing us to avoid use of the non-biodegradable polytetrafluoroethylene (PTFE) fibers. These first results suggest that this technique may prove to be a good model to understand the mechanisms underlying angiogenesis and a useful tool to introduce genetic material into a mammalian host.

In conclusion, these last years have demonstrated that the use of collagen-based biomaterials is still expanding in new application areas defined by the converging fields of biotechnology and biomaterials.

Acknowledgements

The authors acknowledge Coletica (Lyon, France) for the kind supply of collagen biomaterials.

Work in the author's laboratory is supported in part by a BIOMED 2 cont act n° BMH4-CT93–0396 and by a Rhône-Alpes Région grant "Emergence, Sciences de la Vie et de la Santé".

References

Auger FA, Lopez Valle CA, Guignard R, Tremblay N, Noel B, Goulet F, Germain L. Skin equivalent produced with human collagen. In Vitro Cell Dev Biol 1995; 31: 432–9.

Bell E. Deterministic models for tissue engineering. Cell Eng 1995; 28–34.

Bell E, Ehrlich HP, Buttle DJ, Nakatsuji T. Living tissue formed *in vitro* and accepted as skin equivalent tissue of full thickness. Science 1981; 211: 1052–4.

Boyce ST, Christianson DJ, Hansbrough JF. Structure of a collagen-GAG dermal skin substitute optimized for cultured human epidermal keratinocytes. J Biomed Mater Res 1988; 22: 939–57.

Brittberg M, Lindahl A, Nilsson A, Ohlsson C, Isaksson O, Peterson L. Treatment of deep cartilage defects in the knee with autologous chondrocyte transplantation. New Engl J Med 1994; 14: 879–95.

Brown JC, Timpl R. The collagen superfamily. Int Arch Allergy Immunol 1995; 107: 484–90.

Burgeson RE, Nimni ME. Collagen types. Molecular structure and distribution. Clin Orthop Rel Res 1992; 282: 250–72.

Chu CR, Coutts RD, Yoshioka M, Harwood FL, Monosov AZ, Amiel D. Articular cartilage repair using allogeneic perichondrocyte-seeded biodegradable porous polylactic acid (PLA): a tissue-engineering study. J Biomed Mater Res. 1995; 29: 1147–54.

de Vries HJC, Middelkoop E, van Heemstra-Hoen M, Wildevur CHR, Westerhof W. Stromal cells from subcutaneous adipose tissue seeded in a native collagen/elastin dermal substitute reduce wound contraction in a full thickness skin defects. Lab Invest 1995; 73: 532–40.

Doillon CJ, Silver FH, Berg RA. Fibroblast growth on a porous collagen sponge containing hyaluronic acid and fibronectin. Biomaterials 1987; 8: 195–200.

Frondoza C, Sohrabi A, Hungerford D. Human chondrocytes proliferate and produce matrix components in microcarrier suspension culture. Biomaterials 1996; 17: 879–88.

Fujisato T, Sajiki T, Liu Q, Ikada Y. Effect of basic fibroblast growth factor on cartilage regeneration in chondrocytes-seeded collagen sponge scaffold. Biomaterials 1996; 17: 155–62.

Green H, Kehinde O, Thomas J. Growth of cultured human epidermal cells into multiple epithelia suitable for grafting. Proc Nat Acad Sci 1979; 76: 5665–8.

Gumbiner BM. Cell adhesion: the molecular basis of tissue architecture and morphogenesis. Cell 1996; 84: 345–57.

Juliano RL, Haskill S. Signal transduction from the extracellular matrix. J Cell Biol 1993; 120: 577–85.

Koide M, Osaki K, Konishi J, Oyamada K, Katakura T, Takahashi A, Yoshizato K. A new type of biomaterial for artificial skin: dehydrothermally cross-linked composites of fibrillar and denatured collagens. J Biomed Mater Res. 1993; 27: 79–87.

Kühn K, Eble J. The structural bases of integrin-ligand interactions. Trends Cell Biol 1994; 4: 256–61.

Langer R, Vacanti JP. Tissue engineering. Science 1993; 260: 920–926.

Miyata T, Taira T, Noishiki Y. Collagen engineering for biomaterial use. Clinical Materials 1992; 9: 139–48.

Moullier P, Bohl D, Heard JM, Danos O. Correction of lysosomal storage in the liver and spleen of MPS VII mice by implantation of genetically modified skin fibroblasts. Nature Genet 1993; 4: 154–9.

Moullier P, Bohl D, Cardoso J, Heard JM, Danos O. Long-term delivery of a lysosomal enzyme by genetically modified fibroblast in dogs. Nature Med 1995; 1: 353–7.

Nixon AJ, Sams AE, Lust G, Grande D, Mohammed HO. Temporal matrix synthesis and histologic features of a chondrocyte-laden porous collagen cartilage analogue. Amer J Vet Res 1993; 54: 349–56.

Olde Damink LHH. Structure and properties of cross-linked dermal sheep collagen. PhD thesis, University of Twente, 1993.

Petite H, Rault I, Huc A, Menasche Ph, Herbage D. Use of the acyl azide method for cross-linking collagen-rich tissues such as pericardium. J Biomed Mater Res 1990; 24: 179–87.

Petite H, Frei V, Huc A, Herbage D. Use of diphenylphosphoryl azide for cross-linking collagen-based biomaterials. J Biomed Mater Res 1994; 28: 159–65.

Petite H, Duval JL, Frei V, Abdul-Malak N, Sigot-Luizard MF, Herbage D. Cytocompatibility of calf pericardium treated by glutaraldehyde and by the acyl azide methods in an organotypic culture model. Biomaterials 1995; 16: 1003–8.

Prockop DJ, Kivirikko KI. Collagens: molecular biology, diseases, and potentials for therapy. Annu Rev Biochem 1995; 64: 403–34.

Prunieras M. To reconstitute skin: theme and variations. Matrix 1991; 11: 302–5.

Rault I, Frei V, Herbage D, Abdul-Malak N, Huc A. Evaluation of different chemical methods for cross-linking collagen gel, films and sponges. J Mater Sci Mater in Med 1996; 7: 215–21.

Reddi AH. Symbiosis of biotechnology and biomaterials: applications in tissue engineering of bone and cartilage. J Cell Biochem 1994; 56: 192–5.

Sabelman EF. Biology, biotechnology and biocompatibility of collagen, in: Biocompatibility of tissue analogs. Williams DF Ed., CRC Press, Boca Raton 1985; pp 28–66.

Shahabeddin L, Berthod F, Damour O, Collombel C. Characterisation of skin reconstructed on a chitosan-cross-linked collagen glycosaminoglycan matrix. Skin Pharmacol 1990; 3: 107–14.

Sittinger M, Reitzel D, Daumer M, Hierlemann H, Hammer C, Kastenbauer E, Planck H, Burmester GR, Bujía J. Resorbable polyesters in cartilage engineering: affinity and biocompatibility of polymer fiber structures to chondrocytes. J Biomed Mater Res Appl. Biomat 1996; 33: 57–63.

Suzuki S, Matsuda K, Isshiki N, Tamada Y, Yoshioka K, Ikada Y. Clinical evaluation of a new bilayer artificial skin composed of collagen sponge and silicone layer. Brit J Plast Surg 1990; 43: 47–54.

Thomson JA, Haudenschild CC, Anderson KD, Dipietro JM, French Anderson W, Maciag T. Heparin-binding growth factor 1 induces the formation of organoid neovascular structures *in vivo*. Proc Natl Acad Sci 1989; 86: 7928–32.

Toolan BC, Frenkel SR, Pachence JM, Yalowitz L, Alexander H. Effects of growth-factor-enhanced culture on a chondrocyte-collagen implant for cartilage repair. J Biomed Mater Res 1996; 31: 273–80.

Tuckwell DS, Humphries MJ. Molecular and cellular biology of integrins. Crit Rev Oncol/Hematol 1993; 15: 149–71.

van der Rest M, Garrone R, Herbage D. Collagen, a family of proteins with many facets. Adv Mol Cell Biol 1993; 6: 1–67.

van Wachem PB, van Luyn MJA, Olde Damink LHH, Dijkstra PJ, Feijen J, Nieuwenhuis P. Biocompatibility and tissue regenerating capacity of cross-linked dermal sheep collagen. J Biomed Mater Res 1994; 28: 353–63.

Werkmeister JA, Ramshaw JAM. Collagen-based biomaterials. Clinical Materials 1992; 9: 137–8.

Yannas IV. Biologically active analogues of the extracellular matrix: artificial skin and nerves. Angew Chem Int Ed Engl 1990; 29: 20–35.

Yannas IV, Burke JF. Design of an artificial skin. I. Basic design principles. J Biomed Mater Res 1980; 14: 65–81.

The Effect of Gentamicin, Bacterial Infection, and Different Irrigation Solutions on Cartilage Metabolism of the Rat

Results of *in vitro* and *in vivo* animal studies

S. K. Bulstra, R. J. Wolvius, R. Kuijer, G. H. I. M. Walenkamp, N. H. M. Hoefnagels, R. van den Munckhof

Introduction

Bacterial joint infections cause rapid cartilage destruction and loss of function (Curtiss, 1969; Daniel, 1973; Kelly, 1977; Phemister, 1924; Salter, 1981; Smith, 1987). Despite early diagnosis and aggressive surgical drainage combined with appropriate intravenous antibiotic treatment, considerable proteoglycan loss from the cartilage matrix is seen, resulting in continuing destruction of the cartilage (Editorial, 1986; Gillespie, 1987; Nade, 1987; Riegels-Nilesen, 1987; Smith, 1987). Experiments by others showed that even after vigorous washing, although it is usually the first step in therapy, large numbers of bacteria remained adhered to the cartilage surface and penetrated into the non-vascularized cartilage matrix, where they are more difficult to reach for intravenously administered antibiotics (Nade, 1987).

Septic arthritis occurs specially in patients with reduced capacity to eliminate bacterial organisms (children, elderly, immune-compromised patients). Relatively toxic broad-spectrum antibiotics have to be used until bacterial culture and sensitivity results are available. These antibiotics may cause a range of systemic side-effects in these already vulnerable patients (Brummet, 1978; Jackson, 1971; Mannion, 1981; Sensi, 1980). The effectivity of antibiotic treatment is also dependent on the penetration of the drug into the joint space and the surrounding tissue. In general, good penetration of antibiotics into the joint space and the cartilage are found (Baciocco, 1971; Dee, 1977; Howell, 1972; Marsh, 1974; Schurman, 1975). However, considerable inter- and intra-patient differences in drug concentration and a decrease in drug concentration with duration of the disease complicate the effective treatment of the disease (Frimondt-Moller, 1987; Sattar, 1983; Schurmann, 1975).

With regard to the good results achieved with local treatment of osteomyelitis (Buchholz, 1981; Walenkamp, 1988), the intra-articular administration of antibiotics might also be beneficial in the treatment of bacterial arthritis, ensuring high local antibiotic concentrations without the generation of serious general side-effects. Local delivery systems containing gentamicin, such as bone cement and gentamicin-containing collagen, have acquired wide acceptance in the local treatment of bone infections (Walenkamp, 1988). However, the effect of these carriers containing gentamicin on cartilage metabolism has not been studied thoroughly yet.

Therefore, the present studies were undertaken to determine the effect of high doses of gentamicin on cartilage metabolism *in vitro* on rat patella explants. Also, the effect of different irrigation solutions on rat patella metabolism was studied *in vivo* as well as the effect of hyaluronic acid on the already deteriorated cartilage metabolism. The latest experiments looked into the effect of locally aplied Garacol versus sham and non-operated rat knees *in vivo*.

In vitro Studies in the Rat

Materials and Methods

Sampling of patellae: Male, 12–14-week-old Lewis rats were used for these experiments. The rats were sacrificed using ether anesthesia, followed by cervical dislocation. Whole patellae were carefully dissected from the surrounding soft tissue. In total 42 rats were used for these experiments. Seventy-eight patellae were used for the measurement of ^{35}S-sulfate incorporation and another 6 patellae for histological evaluation, having been exposed to different concentrations of gentamicin for 6 or 8 hours, respectively.

Culture technique: After isolation, the patellae were transferred to culture disks, containing 3 ml of M199 culture medium (Gibco, Paisley, Scotland) supplemented with 10% fetal calf serum (FCS, Boehringer, Mannheim, Germany), 250 µg/ml L-glutamine, and 50 µg/ml ascorbic acid. The patellae were cultured at 37 degrees Celsius in a humidified atmosphere of 5 % CO_2 in air for a preincubation time of two hours. Culture medium was changed every 24 hours.

Experimental protocol: After a preincubation period of two hours at 37 °C under 5 % CO_2 in humidified air, all 84 patellae were transferred to fresh medium, with six different concentrations of gentamicin (0, 2, 7, 16, 30, and 50 µg/ml). The incubation was then continued for an additional 6 or 48 hours. Each experimental group consisted of seven patellae; 78 patellae were, after having been rinsed, pre-incubated with clean medium for two hours and subsequently labeled with ^{35}S-sulfate; 6 patellae were used for histology.

For the experiments with the irrigation fluids, 12 patellae were incubated for one hour in the following solutions: Betadine, Ringer's solution, Ringer's lactate, Ringer's glucose, normal saline, and Medium M199. Thereafter a recuperation period of one hour in culture medium M199 was allowed before radiolabeling started.

Histology: After incubation with 50 µg/ml gentamicin for 48 hours, 6 whole patellae were fixed in cold 4 % neutral buffered formalin for 24 hours, whereafter the tissue was rinsed. The patellae were subsequently demineralized in 5 % formic acid for 48 hours and dehydrated in a series of ethanol solutions. Five micrometer sections were cut perpendicular to the surface and mounted on glass slides, then stained with safranin-O fast green, thionin, and alcian blue PAS. For the histo-pathologic score of the cartilage a modification of a procedure originally proposed by Mankin et al. (Bulstra, 1989; Kiviranta, 1985; Mankin, 1971) was used.

Metabolic study: The synthesis of glycosaminoglycans (GAG) was measured by the specific incorporation of ^{35}S-sulfate (Radiochemical Center, Amersham, United Kingdom): 78 patellae were labeled for 16 hours with 5 µCi/ml $Na_2{}^{35}SO_4$ (specific activity, 38 mCi/mmol) after a preincubation period in clean culture medium for two hours.

After labeling the patellae were washed three times in PBS and rinsed in water, to remove most of the non-incorporated label. In 72 patellae the cartilage was removed from the subchondral bone and subsequently digested with protease K (2.5 U in 1 ml 0.05 M tris-HCl, 1 mM $CaCl_2$, Ph 7.9)

at 63 °C for 6 hours. In 6 patellae the whole patella was digested in order to determine the amount of ^{35}S-sulfate that was confined to the bone matrix. The amount of ^{35}S-sulfate incorporated in the GAG of the patellae was determined with a liquid scintillation counter (Beckmann LS 3801).

Pharmacological analysis: Concentrations ranging from 0 to 50 µg/ml of gentamicin in incubation medium were used. The final concentration of gentamicin *in vitro* was determined just before starting each *in vitro* radioactive labeling experiment. The protein binding of gentamicin was determined in the culture medium M199 supplemented with 10 % FCS, using a fluorescence polarized immuno assay (FPIA, E.M.I.T., SYVA, Amsterdam, The Netherlands).

Results

Drug concentration: In this study we used gentamicin concentrations ranging from 0 to 50 µg/ml. The concentrations measured just before the addition of radioactive label were in agreement with the titrated concentrations at the beginning of the experiment. Our data showed that gentamicin in our culture system was not protein bound, which means that the total gentamicin fraction matches the free gentamicin fraction.

Histology: For the histo-pathologic grading of the patellae exposed to gentamicin, we used the modified Mankin score. No loss of stainability of cartilage matrix was seen when we examined the sections with specific stains such as safranin-O, thionin, and alcian blue. It appeared that cartilage structure and chondrocyte morphology were unaffected by gentamicin.

In the study with the irrigating solutions only the patellae that were treated with betadine showed clear softening of the cartilage. Histologically for the other irrigation solutions no clear cartilage breakdown could be demonstrated.

Metabolic study: In this study the effect of gentamicin on the metabolic capacity of chondrocytes in anatomically intact isolated rat patellae was assessed. The patellae were cultured for a short period, in order to prevent leakage of GAG into the culture medium. We found that 98 % of the radiolabel was confined to the cartilage layer of the patella and 2 % to the subchondral bone, while the interindividual weight difference of the patellae was minimal (de Vries, 1986). The

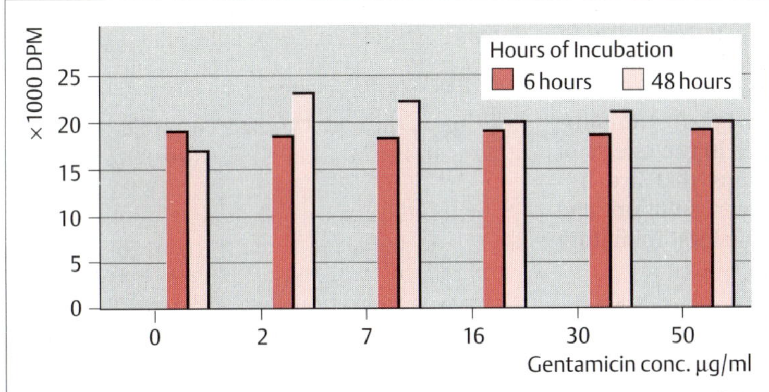

Fig. 1   Effect of gentamicin on cartilage metabolism.

^{35}S-sulfate incorporation was used to quantify the GAG synthesis. Our data showed that even high concentrations of gentamicin did not inhibit the GAG synthesis of these patellae *in vitro*. After 6 hours exposure of the patellae to different gentamicin concentrations, no significant changes in chondrocyte metabolism were seen. Even after prolonged exposure to gentamicin (48 hrs), cartilage metabolism was not inhibited (Fig. **1**).

In the experiments with the irrigating solutions it was shown that the saline and the Ringer's lactate inhibited significantly cartilage metabolism by 20% ($p < 0.001$). Ringer's solution and Ringer glucose showed an inhibition of metabolism by 10% ($p < 0.01$). Betadine served as the positive control and showed an inhibition of metabolism by 55% ($p < 0.001$) when compared to culture medium (Fig. **2**).

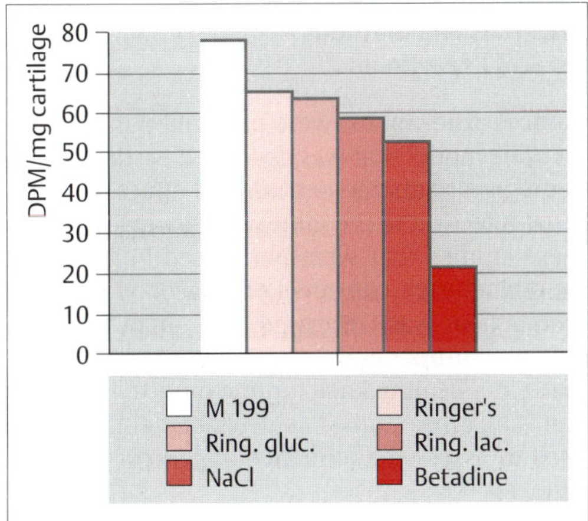

Fig. **2**   Effect of different irrigating solutions on cartilage metabolism.

Discussion

The analysis of the effect of gentamicin on the metabolism of the patella was assessed using $Na_2{}^{35}SO_4$ incorporation in the GAG. ^{35}S-sulfate incorporation into the GAG has been shown to be a good marker of cartilage metabolism (Sandy, 1980; Vries, 1986). Our data showed that even after 48 hours of incubation, the metabolism of the chondrocytes was not inhibited by gentamicin up to a dose of 50 µg/ml.

Pharmacological analysis revealed that in our culture system gentamicin was not bound to serum protein, which might be in contrast to the *in vivo* situation (Howell, 1972). The effective free drug concentration was therefore very high and in correspondence with the actual drug concentration used.

The effect of irrigation solution on cartilage metabolism was studied because in most cases where an arthritis is present, next to antibiotic treatment, an extensive debridement of the joint is performed. Also, we were interested in the effects of different irrigation solutions used frequently during arthroscopy of the joints. Our data show that all of the irrigation solutions tested had an inhibitory effect when compared to short-term *in vitro* culture of the patella in culture medium. Although other authors consider articular chondrocytes to be capable of a quick recovery (Arciero et al., 1986), we showed definite inhibition of metabolism after a recovery time of 16 hours with a prolonged exposure to the radiolabel.

In conclusion our data suggest that the intra-articular administration of gentamicin is not impeding on healthy cartilage metabolism, although a high concentration of the antibiotic is present inside the cartilage. Therefore it seems likely that gentamicin administrated intra-articulary directly after the onset of a joint infection is useful in the treatment of the infection, while not being harmful to the cartilage. At the same time, there is quite a difference in the effects of the different irrigation solutions that are frequently used clinically. Ringer's solution and Ringer glucose seem to have the least inhibitory effects in these *in vitro* studies.

In vivo Animal Studies

As a consequence of the results of these *in vitro* studies we decided to perform some *in vivo* studies exploring the effects of the irrigating solution in conjunction with hyaluronic acid in the rat knee. Also Garacol as one of the new gentamicin carriers was examined in the rabbit knee, to explore its effect on cartilage metabolism using histological and metabolic tools.

Materials and Methods – Hyaluronic Acid Experiments

In this study the rabbit knee was used *in vivo*. The knees of the rabbit were irrigated with saline of which we already know that it has an inhibiting effect on cartilage metabolism. In total, both knees were irrigated with 5 ml of saline in twelve rabbits. After irrigation, different concentrations of hyaluronic acid upto 10 mg/ml were instilled in the knee, with a volume of 0.5 ml. In six rabbits hyaluronic acid in a concentration of 5 mg/ml was used as an **irrigation solution** in order to study the effect on knee cartilage metabolism.

Results

The results are shown in Fig. **3**. As a control M199 was used in 4 rabbits. The results from left to right show that irrigation with 5 mg/ml hyaluronic acid showed a non-significant and slight inhibition of cartilage metabolism after two days, while when metabolism was measured after 7 days also no statistically important inhibition was found. Irrigation with NaCl showed a clear and statistically significant inhibition of cartilage metabolism, when measured 2 or 7 days after the irrigation procedure.

One injection with 5 mg/ml hyaluronic acid after irrigation of the knee with 5 ml NaCl, was able to restore the cartilage metabolism when measured two and seven days after the procedure (p < 0.01).

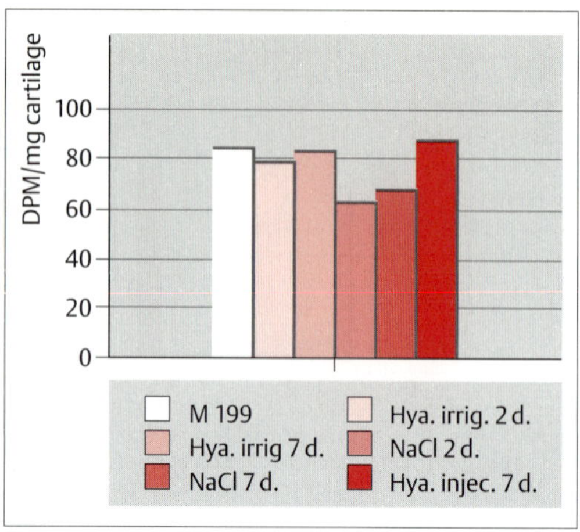

Fig. **3** Effect of hyaluronic acid on cartilage metabolism.

Discussion

In this study it was proven that not only *in vitro* but also *in vivo* NaCl had a clear inhibitory effect on cartilage metabolism. Irrigation with hyaluronic acid did not have this inhibiting effect which is supported by many *in vitro* and *in vivo* studies that were performed by others. It is surprising that only one injection of hyaluronic acid (5 mg/ml), after irrigation of the knee with NaCl, was able to restore the inhibited cartilage metabolism, when measured 2 and 7 days after the experiment. The reason for this result might be found in the restoration at least in part of the normal viscosity of the synovial fluid.

Materials and Methods – Garacol Experiments

Garacol experiments were performed in the rabbit knee model that was described earlier. In earlier experiments the detrimental effect of a bacterial infection to the joint was shown (Fig. **4**). In these studies that were performed in groups of six rabbits each, the effect of garacol on cartilage metabolism was compared to a sham-operated and a non-operated knee. Garacol was left in place in a healthy knee for one month. Histology and radiolabel studies as described earlier were used to assess the influence of garacol on cartilage.

Judgement observers 1 and 2		Medial condyle	Trochlea
Garacol vs. sham	1	p < 0.141	p < 0.417
	2	p < 0.052*	p < 0.908
Garacol vs. Non-operated	1	p < 0.196	p < 0.049*
	2	p < 0.039*	p < 0.430
Sham vs. Non-operated	1	p < 0.813	p < 0.197
	2	p < 0.817	p < 0.506

Table 1 Histology by the modified Mankin score

The table shows the histological effect of Garacol vs. non- and sham-operated knee of the rabbit. Two observers have independently scored using the modified Mankin score.
* gives a significant negative effect on cartilage histology for the first of the two treatments.

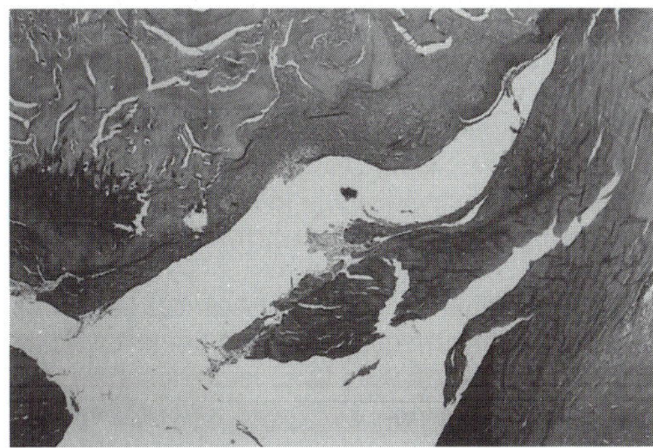

Fig. **4** Effect of Garacol on rabbit knee.

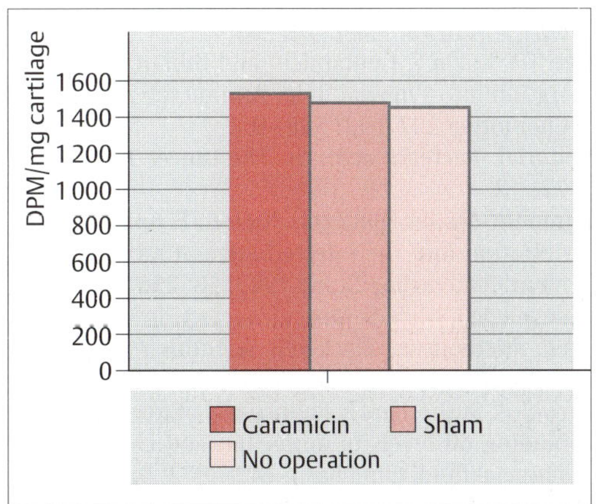

Fig. **5** Effect of Garacol versus sham- and non-operated knee.

Results

In histological sections stained with safranin-O fast green and Alcian blue the modified Mankin score was applied double blind, by two different observers. The data show (Table **1**) that some slight differences in the histological quality were found in the medial condyle in the garacol vs sham and versus the non-operated knee, by one of the two observers.

Metabolic data, however, did not show a statistically important influence of Garacol on cartilage metabolism (Fig. **5**).

Discussion

Although one observer found a slightly decreased result in the modified Mankin score in the medial condyle, this conclusion was not supported by the other observer, nor for the trochlea by both observers. The data given are the result of a statistical analysis for a difference of one point on the Mankin scale. When we, however, used a difference of two points on this scale, the difference in score and the influence of Garacol on cartilage metabolism proved not to be of statistical importance. In the literature it is found that even highly trained and experienced observers produce scores for the same material with a standard deviation of two. We suppose therefore that in reality the differences in Mankin score found in this study fall within the standard deviation of the measurement by two observers.

The results of the metabolic study seem to warrant this conclusion, because no significant influence of Garacol on cartilage metabolism could be found in this study. These results are supported by the results of the *in vitro* study presented earlier in this article.

We conclude, therefore, that gentamicin or gentamicin embedded in a collagen carrier (Garacol) did not clearly influence cartilage metabolism in this *in vivo* animal study.

References

Arciero RA, Little JS, Liebenberg SP, Parr TJ. Irrigation solutions used in arthroscopy and their effect on articular cartilage: an *in vivo* study. Orthopaedics 1989; 9: 1511 – 15.

Baciocco EA, Iles RL. Ampicillin and kanamycin concentrations in joint fluid. Clin Pharmacol and Ther 1971; 12: 858 – 63.

Bailleu E, Paul B, Koch P. Auswirkungen einmaliger intraartikulärer Antibiotikagaben auf die Knorpelstruktur beim Kaninchen. Z exp Chir transplant 1987; 2: 94 – 8.

Brummet RE, Fox KE, Bendrick FW, Himes DC. Ototoxicity of tobramycin, gentamicin, amikacin and sisomycin in the guinea pig. J of Antimicr Chemoth 1978; 4: 73 – 9.

Buchholz HW, Elson RA, Engelbrecht E, Lodenkamper H, Rottger J, Siegel A. Management of deep infection of total hip replacement. J Bone Joint Surg (Br) 1981; 63-B: 342 – 53.

Bulstra SK, Buurman WA, Walenkamp GHIM, Linden van der AJ. Metabolic characteristics of *in vitro* cultured human chondrocytes in relation to the histopathologic grade of osteoarthritis. Clin Orthop Rel Res 1989; 242: 294 – 302.

Bulstra SK, Kuijer R, Eerdmans P, van der Linden AJ. The effect *in vitro* of irrigating solutions on intact rat articular cartilage. J Bone Joint Surg 1994; Vol 76-B, No 3: 468 – 9.

Curtiss PH. Cartilage damage in septic arthritis. Clin Orthop Rel Res 1969; 64: 87 – 90.

Daniel D, Boyer J, Green S, Amiel D, Akeson W. Cartilage destruction in experimentally produced *Staphylococcus aureus* joint infection: *in vivo* study. Surg Forum 1973; 24: 479 – 81.

Dee TH, Kozin F. Gentamicin and tobramycin penetration into synovial fluid. Antimicrob Agents and Chemother 1977; 12: 548 – 9.

Editorial: Bacterial arthritis. The Lancet 1986; Sept: 721 – 2.

Frimondt-Moller N, Riegels-Nielsen P. Antibiotic penetration into the infected knee. A rabbit experiment. Acta orthop Scand 1987; 58: 256 – 9.

Gillespie WJ, Nade S. Musculoskeletal infections. 1st ed., Melbourne: Blackwell Scientific Publications 1987: 290 – 3.

Howell A, Sutherland R, Rolinson GN. Effect of protein binding on levels of ampicillin and cloxacillin in synovial fluid. Clin Pharm Ther 1972; 5: 724 – 32.

Jackson GG, Arcieri G. Ototoxicity of gentamicin in man: a survey and controled analysis of clinical experience in the united states. J Inf Dis 1971; 124: 130 – 5.

Kelly PJ. Infections of bones and joints in adult patients. Instructional course lectures 1977, Vol 36, Mosley, St. Louis, chapter 1: 3 – 13.

Kiviranta NI, Jurvelin J, Tammi M, Helminen HI. Microspectrophotometric quantitation of glycosaminoglycans in articular cartilage sections stained with safranin-O. Histochem. J. 1985; 82: 249–55.

Mankin HJ, Dorfman H, Lipiello MS, Zarins A. Biochemical and metabolic abnormalities in articular cartilage from osteo-arthritic human hips. J Bone Joint Surg (Am) 1971; 53-A: 523–37.

Mannion JC, Bloch R, Popovich NG. Cephalosporin-aminoglycoside synergistic nephrotoxicity: fact or fiction? Drug Intell and Clin Pharmacy 1981; 15: 248–52.

Marsh DC, Matthew EB, Persellin RH. Transport of gentamicin into synovial fluid. JAMA 1974; 228: 607.

Nade S, Speers DJ. Staphylococcal adherence to chicken cartilage. Acta Orthop Scand 1987; 58: 351–353.

Phemister DB. The effect of pressure on articular surfaces in pyogenic and tuberculous arthritides and its bearing on treatment. Ann Surg 1924; 80: 484–500.

Riegels-Nilesen P, Frimondt-Moller N, Jensen JS. Rabbit model of septic arthritis. Acta Orthop Scand 1987; 58: 14–9.

Rosenberg L. Chemical basis for histological use of safranin-O in the study of articular cartilage. J Bone Joint Surg 1971; 53-A: 69–82.

Salter RB, Bell RS, Keeley FW. The protective effect of continuous passive motion on living articular cartilage in acute septic arthritis. Clin Orthop Rel Res 1981; 159: 224–47.

Sandy JD, Brown HLG, Lowther DA. Control of proteoglycan synthesis. Studies on the activation of synthesis observed during culture of articular cartilages. Biochem J 1980; 188: 119–30.

Sattar MA, Barratt SP, Cawley ID. Concentrations of some antibiotics in synovial fluid after oral administration, with special reference to antistaphylococcal activity. Ann Rheum Dis 1983; 42: 67–74.

Schurman DJ, Johnson BL, Finerman G, Amstutz HC. Antibiotic bone penetration; Concentrations of methicillin and clindamycin phosphate in human bone taken during total hip replacement. Clin Orthop Rel Res 1975; 111: 142–146.

Schurman DJ, Hirshman HP, Nagel DA. Antibiotic penetration of synovial fluid in infected and normal knee joints. Clin Orth Rel Res 1978; 136: 304–10.

Sensi M, Pozzili P, Cattell WR. Gentamicin nephrotoxicity in experimental acute renal failure. Acta ther 1980; 6: 65–8.

Smith RL, Merchant TC, Schurman DJ. *In vitro* cartilage degradation by *Escherichia coli* and *Staphylococcus aureus*. Arthritis Rheum 1982; Vol 25, No 4: 441–6.

Smith RL, Schurman DJ, Kajiyama G, Bell M, Gilkerson E. The effect of antibiotics on the destruction of cartilage in experimental infectious arthritis. J Bone Joint Surg (Am) 1987; 69-A: 1063–8.

Vries de BJ, Berg van den WB, Vitters E, Putte von de LBA. Quantitation of glycosaminoglycan metabolism in anatomically intact articular cartilage of the mouse patella: *in vitro* and *in vivo* studies with ^{35}S-sulfate, ^{3}H-glucosamine and ^{3}H-acetate. Rheumatol Int 1986; 6: 273–81.

Walenkamp GHIM, Vree TB, Rens van TJG. Gentamicin-PMMA beads. Pharmacokinetic and nephrotoxicologcial study. Clin Orthop Rel Res 1988; 205: 171–83.

Pharmacokinetics of two Gentamicin Collagen Fleeces in Animal Experiments

G. H. I. M. Walenkamp, R. J. Wolvius S. Kaarsemaker

Introduction

Gentamicin PMMA beads must be removed when they are not needed any more, mostly after two weeks of implantation. This operation for removal can be combined with reconstructive measures (e.g., bone graft, reimplantation of prosthesis) or with a repeated debridement if healing was not adequate. Resorbable antibiotic carriers can make the operation for removal unnecessary. Another advantage of some resorbable antibiotic carriers is that they can be put in places where no room is left for large beads or minibeads, and they also have the possibility to admix them in bone grafts or bone substitutes.

Gentamicin collagen fleeces have been developed on the basis of the experience gained with plain collagen as used for local hemostasis in surgery. Collagen is characterized by good tolerance and complete dissolution by phagocytosis and enzymatic degradation. Admixture of gentamicin in a collagen fleece results in a release of the gentamicin in days or weeks. There are two commercial products composed of gentamicin collagen fleeces.

The first to be developed was a collagen fleece (Ascherl et al., 1986) marketed by Schering Plough (Sulmycin®, Gentacoll®, Garacoll®, or Garamycin®). This collagen fleece has a size of $10 \times 10 \times 0.5$ cm. The fleece is white, contains 280 mg of collagen type I from bovine tendons and 200 mg of gentamicin sulfate, equivalent to 130 mg of gentamicin base.

The second fleece was developed in the laboratories of E. Merck, Darmstadt (EMD 53155, Septocoll®). This fleece is yellow, the size is $8 \times 5 \times 0.3$ cm and contains 461 mg of bovine skin collagen. The fleece contains two kinds of gentamicin: the regular hydrophilic gentamicin sulfate, and a newly developed hydrophobic gentamicin crobophate, a flavanoid form of gentamicin. The gentamicin crobophate will slowly undergo decomposition into a phosphate and flava-

nol, which results in a more protracted release of the gentamicin. In one fleece the total amount of gentamicin is equivalent to 70 mg of gentamicin base.

At our department both types of gentamicin fleeces were studied in animal experiments with particular attention to pharmacokinetics, safety, and effectivity. We present here some of the preliminary results on the pharmacokinetics.

Garacol® Fleeces in Septic Arthritis in Rabbits

In rabbits a septic arthritis was developed. *Staphylococcus aureus* was injected in the knee: 5×10^8 CFU of bacteria (Wolvius, 1996). After two days a debridement of the infection was performed and a quarter of a fleece implanted intra-articularly, equivalent to 32.5 mg of gentamicin base. The gentamicin concentrations were measured in the serum (day 1) and in the tissues of the knee (days 2, 4 and 7) namely in cartilage, bone, meniscus, and synovial tissue.

The serum concentration remained below levels that can be regarded as toxic. The highest level was reached after $1-2$ hours, and was $4-9$ µg/ml. After 24 hours, gentamicin was no longer detectable in the serum (detection level: 0.2 µg/ml).

The tissue concentrations of gentamicin varied largely, but in general showed very high concentrations in all tissues at day two, especially in the cartilage ($750-1350$ µg/g). At day seven these concentrations in the cartilage were still high ($11-42$ µg/g). The concentrations in the synovial tissues showed a pattern parallel to those of the cartilage (Fig. **1**).

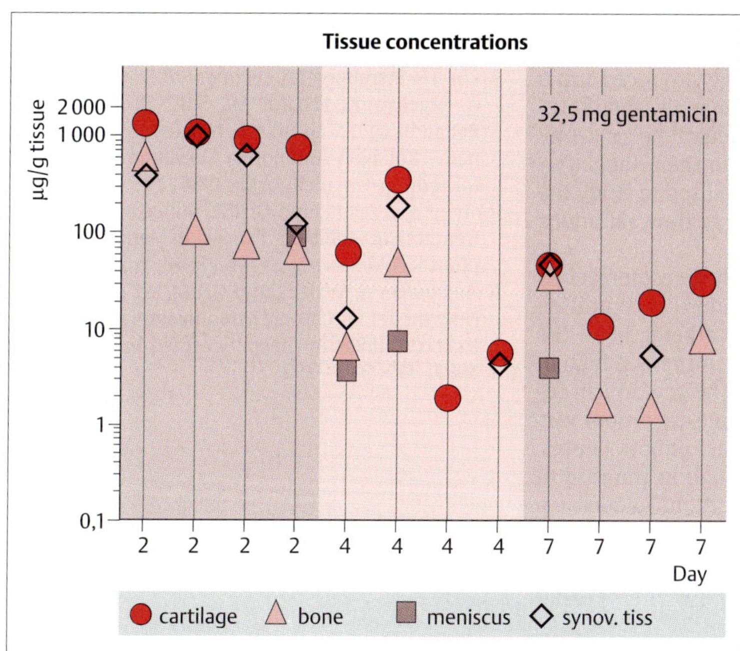

Fig. 1   Garacol in rabbit septic arthritis.

Septocoll® Fleeces in Chronic Osteomyelitis in Sheep

An osteomyelitis model was developed in sheep: 4×10^8 CFU of *Staphylococcus aureus* were soaked in gelatin sponge strips and injected in the proximal metaphysis of the tibia. No corpus alienum was implanted and a chronic osteomyelitis developed in 3 months (Kaarsemaker, 1997). At that time the sheep were operated and a debridement was performed of the localized chronic osteomyelitis. Further treatment consisted of systemic gentamicin antibiotic therapy, comprising gentamicin Septopal® minibeads or Septocoll® gentamicin fleeces. The sheep were sacrified after 3 weeks or 3 months. The serum and urine concentrations of gentamicin were measured during the first 14 days of implantation. The tissue concentrations were determined at 3 weeks or 3 months.

The implanted amount of gentamicin was equivalent to 17 or 34 mg of gentamicin base in case of the 10 or 20 minibeads, and 35 or 70 mg in case of the gentamicin Septocoll® fleeces (one or a half fleece). The pharmacokinetics of the beads and fleeces were compared.

Gentamicin was not detectable in the serum (detectable level 0.2 µg/ml) of any of the sheep treated with beads or fleece. In the urine the ex-

cretion ws high during the first one to two days after implantation in beads as well as in fleeces. The maximum level was higher and was reached earlier postoperatively in the case of implanted fleeces.

The tissue concentrations of gentamicin were measured in the endosteum, three different cortical layers, and the periosteum. The concentration was the highest at the endosteal level at three weeks in the case of beads as well as fleeces, reflecting the gentamicin that is still being released at that moment in the bone marrow. At three months there was still gentamicin detectable in the cortical layers of the bone. In the case of 20 minibeads (N = 5, 34 mg of gentamicin base) we measured 2 – 10 µg/g, and in a case of a half fleece (N = 2, 35 mg of gentamicin base) we found 2 – 7 µg/g of gentamicin in the three different cortical bone layers.

Conclusions

These experiments with beads and with two types of collagen fleeces informed us about the pharmacokinetics in different release carriers. In general, the elution of gentamicin out of the collagen is high in the first postoperative day, resulting in serum concentrations that may be detectable at that moment. When, later on, these serum concentrations are below the detection level, the urine concentration can still provide further information. Collection of all the produced urine can be very difficult in small animals, and therefore urine excretion rates cannot be correctly measured. The concentration in the urine, influenced by the urine flow, can be used to study the release of gentamicin if no large flow variations exist.

In the experiments with sheep osteomyelitis we were able to measure the urine concentration every day, collected by urine catheter. In all the sheep the concentration in the urine was high in the first day postoperatively. The gentamicin release, as expressed in the urine excretion, was higher in the first day in the case of both fleeces, but remained for more days high in the case of beads. In fleeces as well as beads, no gentamicin could be found in the urine after 10–14 days. Thus, the gentamicin still present in the bone after 3 months, must result in a urine excretion below the detection level.

Fleeces can be used to create high local tissue levels of gentamicin in contaminated tissues. The release varies between the different types of fleeces and as compared with beads. Depending of the indications for use, the surgeon could chose between a carrier with a very high release in the first hours, e.g., in case of prophylaxis, or a carrier with a more protracted release, resorbable or not, in case of treatment and reconstructions.

References

Ascherl R, Stemberger A, Lechner F, Plaumann L, Rupp G, Machka K, Erhardt W, Sorg KH, Blumel G. Behandlung der chronischen Osteomyelitis mit einem Kollagen-Antibiotika Verbund. Vorläufige Mitteilung. Unfallchirurgie 1986; 12 (3): 125–7.

Wolvius R, Walenkamp GHIM, Kuijer R, Bulstra SK. Gentamicin collagen fleeces in septic arthritis: pharmacokinetics in a rabbit knee. Submitted.

Kaarsemaker S, Walenkamp GHIM, vd Bogaard AEJ. New model for chronic osteomyelitis with *Staphylococcus aureus* in sheep. Accepted in Clin Orthop 1997; 339: 246–252.

Comparative Human Pharmacokinetics of two Gentamicin-Containing Collagen Carriers

A. Moser

Introduction

Even today infections are a problem in the field of traumatology that should not be underestimated. The basic principle of an adequate surgical treatment of the infection is a radical debridement of all infected and necrotic tissue by means of a possibly primary closure of the wound. This treatment of the tissue and the necessary minimization of all germs are the preconditions for the healing of the wound.

Where the blood supply in the tissue has been obstructed due to infection or operation, a systemic therapy using antibiotics can hardly build up effective local concentrations of antibiotic. The local therapy, however, releases concentrations of the active agent at the place of implantation which can apparently never be achieved by a systemic therapy (Figs. 1 and 2).

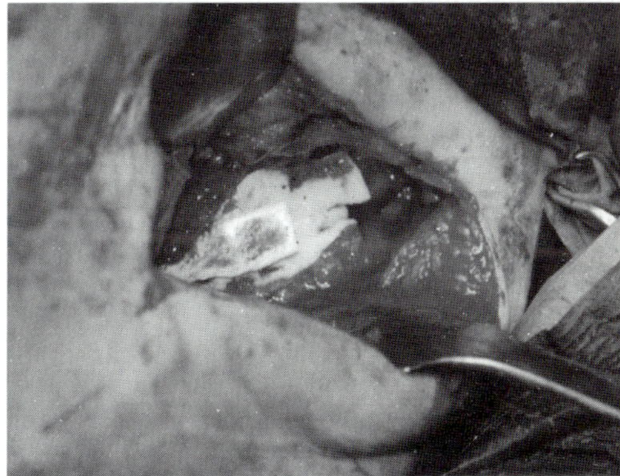

Fig. 2   Placement of gentamicin-collagen-carrier.

tained in samples of serum, wound secretion, and urine at predefined points of time.

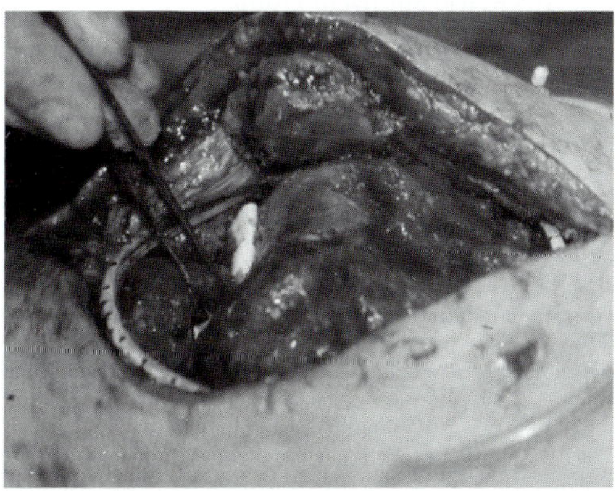

Fig. 1   Implantation of gentamicin-collagen-carrier.

While treating patients for bone infections and bone contaminations, data for the pharmacokinetics of two gentamicin-containing carriers were collected. These data for this prospective and randomized comparative study were ob-

Patients and Methods

Male and female patients aged between 18 and 75 were chosen for this study; they all suffered from bone infection or bone contamination that had been certified by bacteriological and histological tests. The patients were either implanted a Sulmycin sponge or two EMD fleeces.

Samples of serum were taken before and after the operation, six samples on the day of operation and one sample each at 24-hour intervals from the first to the fourth day after the operation. Apart from the pre-operative sample of urine, for the first 10 days after the operation another sample was taken from the urine that had been collected over a period of 24 hours.

As long as there was a flow of secretion out of the overflow drainage, a wound secretion sample was taken after the operation at 0–6 hours, and in the following time, every 24 hours.

In the period from October 1992 to December 1995 there were 40 patients included in the study, 26 male and 14 female. In each of the two groups, there were 13 male and 7 female patients who were treated with the EMD-fleece or the Sulmycin sponge.

The median age in the EMD group was 52 (from 20–76), in the Sulmycin group it was 54 (from 29–80). The patients' height as well as their weight was nearly the same in both groups.

One of the collagen-carriers containing the gentamicin is the Sulmycin implant sponge (size 10 by 10 cm) which has already been on the market for quite some time. Its sole active agent is the soluble gentamicin sulfate in a dose of 200 mg which accounts for a gentamicin base level of 120 mg. The other carrier used in the study was the newly developed test preparation EMD 53 155 (size 8 by 5 cm). As well as the hydrophilous gentamicin sulfate, the EMD fleece contains the newly developed gentamicin crobefate, a hydrophobic gentamicin salt which allows for a protracted release of the active agent (Fig. 3); 70 mg of gentamicin base are equally divided between gentamicin sulfate and gentamicin crobefate.

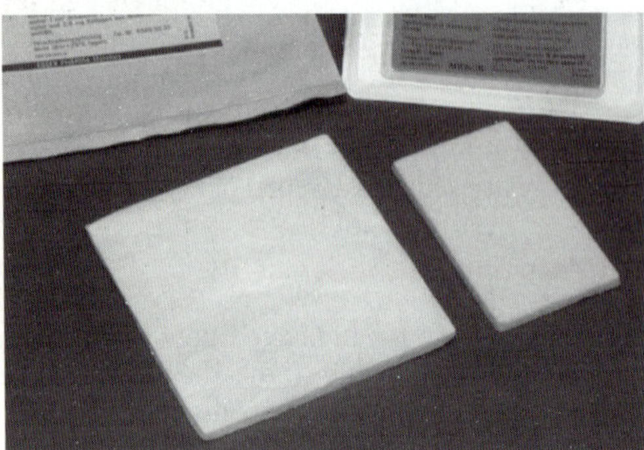

Fig. 3   Sulmycin-sponge/EMD-fleece.

In line with the study design, EMD fleeces 53 155 with a gentamicin base level of 140 mg were used in group A, one Sulmycin implant sponge with a gentamicin base level of 120 mg was used in group B. The different contents of the active agent in the test preparation were corrected by multiplication with the difference (Fig. 4).

The next step now is a direct comparison: the mean values showing the developments of the levels of concentration in serum, urine, and wound secretion are compared.

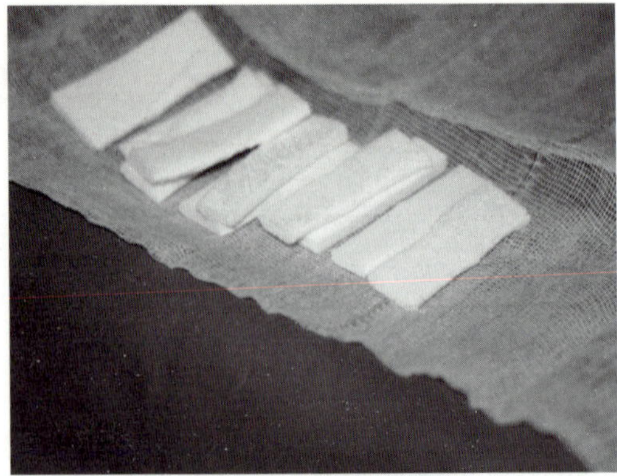

Fig. 4   Preparation before implantation.

Results

When having a look at the median concentration of gentamicin in the serum it becomes apparent for the Sulmycin group that there are significantly higher levels of concentration especially directly after the operation. This value is much higher than the one in the EMD group, where the maximum is at 0.349 µg/ml at 4 hours postoperative. The corresponding value in the Sulmycin group is 0.977 µg/ml at 6 hours postoperative, a value almost three times as high. A stronger scattering of the individual graphs shows the deviations in the Sulmycin group.

A direct comparison of the median values of the gentamicin serum concentration (Fig. 5) shows that the values in the Sulmycin group are much higher for the measuring points 1–24 hours. Even without having corrected the concentrations by the difference of the various gentamicin values, the median values of the measuring points up to 24 hours remain almost twice as high in the Sulmycin group as in the EMD group. Measurement after 24 hours showed that the curves were more and more brought into line.

The AUC values which had been gained from the different concentrations of gentamicin in the serum also show clear differences for the absorption of the gentamicin in the wound area: especially in the period of time 0–24 hours it was 4 689 µg/ml for EMD and 13.35 µg/ml for Sulmycin. These differences decrease at the later measuring times. In both groups a maximum concentration in serum was reached in the first 10 hours after the operation.

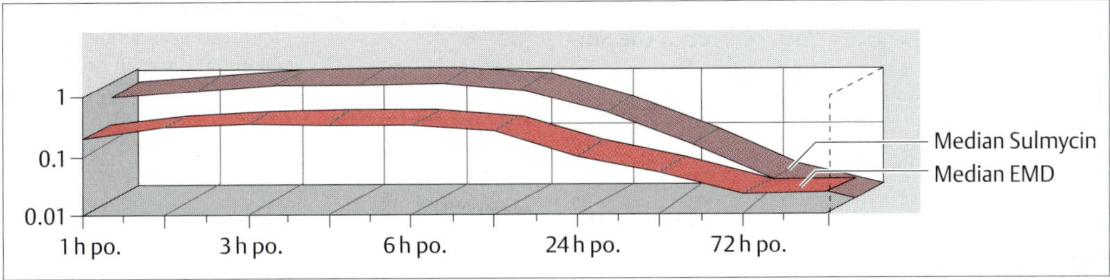

Fig. **5** Gentamicin concentration in serum.

When analyzing the concentration of gentamicin in the wound secretion, relatively strong scatterings become visible for both groups. These differences on the one hand result from the different kinds of implantation (intraosseous, periosseous, in the soft tissue). On the other hand, they can be accounted for by the different ways of obtaining the serum out of one or more drainages.

In the Sulmycin group the first and second days after the operation already showed a concentration of gentamicin lower than 10 µg/ml for 7 out of 16 patients. At the same time the values for all 17 patients in the EMD group were still high, between 60 and 1600 µg/ml. These values could still be measured with 11 out of 14 patients on the third day after the operation.

The median values show the differences in the concentration of gentamicin especially on the third and fourth day after the operation. All in all the median values of the EMD group are without exception higher than those of the Sulmycin group. More constantly and over a longer period of time, high concentrations of gentamicin in the wound secretion are reached in the EMD group because of the protracted release of the active agent.

The gentamicin concentrations in the urine measured in the individual patients of both groups show similar curves without any major differences. The comparison of the mean values, however, reveals that clearly more gentamicin is excreted with the urine in the Sulmycin group.

Especially on the first and second day after the operation the concentration of gentamicin in the urine was almost three times as high in the Sulmycin group as in the EMD group. For the Sulmycin group this means an average excretion of gentamicin of 57.52 mg, i.e., 47.9% of 120 mg. For the EMD group these figures were 45.01 mg, i.e., 32.2% of 140 mg.

A comparison of the maximum concentrations of gentamicin in the wound secretion (Figs. **6** and **7**) shows a relatively homogeneous picture with a relatively high and constant level of gentamicin. The Sulmycin group does show a higher level of gentamicin, but these values are only reached for a short period of time and are subject to greater fluctuations.

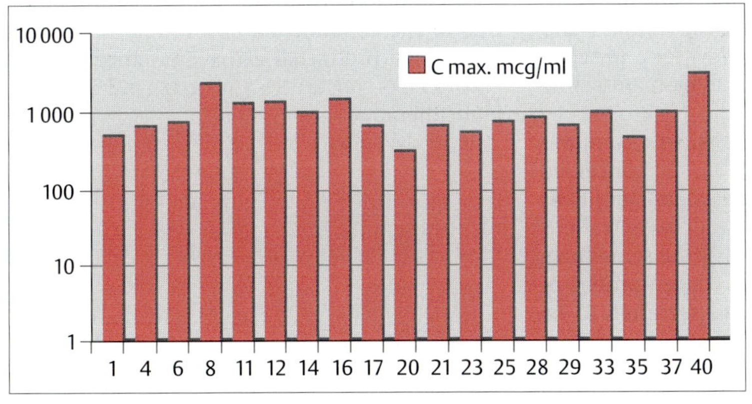

Fig. **6** Gentamicin concentration in wound secretion of EMD group.

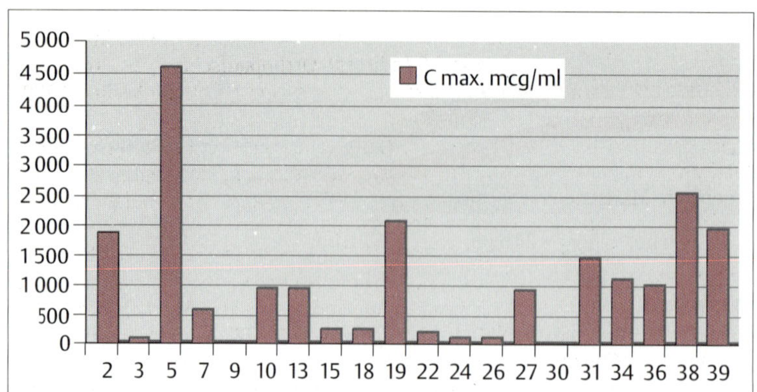

Fig. **7**   Gentamicin concentration in wound secretion of Sulmycin group.

As already shown in the previous median values for the concentration of gentamicin in the serum, the Sulmycin group shows a significantly higher maximum concentration than the EMD group. Both groups, however, did not achieve a continuous level of serum that was higher than 0.2 µg/ml. Thus, a culmulation and any consequent toxic side-effects are not to be expected.

The maximum concentration of gentamicin in the urine did not show any major differences for the two groups. The fluctuation in the Sulmycin group seems to be slightly higher than in the EMD group.

Discussion

Assuming that the effectiveness of a local antibiotic depends on its concentration in the wound secretion and in the surrounding tissue, it can be concluded that local carriers of antibiotics should meet the following requirements when used prophylactically and in the therapy for infections.

Antibiotics that are applied locally should quickly and reliably reach a sufficiently high concentration of the active agent in the wound secretion. Moreover, they should allow for a penetration into the surrounding tissue by maintaining a high level in the tissue.

As a result of this pharmacokinetic comparison of Sulmycin and EMD, it can be concluded that a protracted release of the active agent EMD 53155 leads to lower maximum concentrations and lower levels in the serum. At the same time, however, it allows for higher concentrations of the active agent in the wound secretion to be achieved.

After analyzing the collected data it can be concluded that toxic side-effects caused by gentamicin can be ruled out for both preparations. Considerably lower gentamicin serum concentrations in the EMD group mean increased safety with reference to any side-effects caused by gentamicin when the antibiotic is used in comparable doses.

The median concentrations of gentamicin in the wound secretion are at all times higher in the EMD group than in the Sulmycin group. Therefore, for this preparation an at least equally high antibacterial activity can be expected. Considering an antibacterial effect of EMD that is dependent on its concentration, the high concentrations of gentamicin in the wound secretion after EMD 53155 has been implanted, could be of clinical relevance.

The levels of the active agent that had been aimed at by applying a local antibiotic therapy are reached more reliably in the EMD group than in the Sulmycin group. The EMD 53155 fleece will be available as an adjuvant therapeutic in the treatment of bone and soft-tissue infections. Due to the combination of a locally resorbable carrier and protracted active substance release, EMD 53155 constitutes a progress in local antibiotic therapy.

References

Bethge H, Czechanowski B, Gundert-Remy U, Hasford J, Kleinsorge H, Kreutz G, Letzel H, Müller A, Selbmann HK, Weber E. Empfehlungen zur Ermittlung, Dokumentation, Erfassung und Bewertung unerwünschter Ereignisse im Rahmen der klinischen Prüfung von Arzneimitteln. Im Auftrag der Sektion „Klinische Pharmakologie" der Deutschen Gesellschaft für Pharmakologie und Toxikologie. Arzneim.-Forsch./Drug Res 1989; 39: 1294–1300.10.

Burri C, Rüter A (editors). Lokalbehandlung chirurgischer Infektionen. Aktuelle Probleme in der Chirurgie und Orthopädie, Band 12. Bern: Huber-Verlag, 1979.

Contzen H. Gentamicin-PMMA-chains. Unfallchirurgie, Special Issue, 1977.

De Broe ME, Giuliano RA. Evaluation of the nephrotoxicity of EMD 42 521 (containing 4 g gentamicin) after implantation in chronic renal failure rats. E Merck, Darmstadt, 1988, EMD 42 521–55.

De Broe ME, Giuliano RA. Evaluation of the nephrotoxicity of the gentamicin-containing bone cements: Palacos R and EMD 42 521 after implantation in rats. E. Merck, Darmstadt, 1988, EMD 42 521–56.

Dingeldein E. EMD 53 155 – Gentamicinkonzentrationen in Körperflüssigkeiten von Patienten. E. Merck, Darmstadt, 1990, EMD 53 155–39.

Dingeldein E. Gentamicinkonzentrationen in Körperflüssigkeiten von Patienten nach Implantation von Gentamicin-Kollagen-Vlies in Verbindung mit einer Redondrainage. E. Merck, Darmstadt, 1995, EMD 53 155–67.

Eberle H (editor). Gentamicin-PMMA-Chains in Bone and Soft-Tissue Infections. Basel: Karger-Verlag, 1988.

Grimm H. Bakteriologische und Pharmakokinetische Aspekte der topischen Antibiotikaanwendung. In: Stemberger A, Ascher R, Lechner F, Blümel G, editors. Kollagen als Wirkstoffträger – Einsatzmöglichkeiten in der Chirurgie. Schattauer, Stuttgart, New York 1989: 33–37.

Grove DC, Randall AW. Assay methods of antibiotics. New York: Medical Encyclopedia Inc., 1955. E. Merck, Darmstadt, EMD 53 155–60.

Grüßner U, Langendorff HU, Moser A. Prospektive randomisierte Vergleichsstudie zur Erhebung pharmakokinetischer und klinischer Daten bei Anwendung zweier Gentamicinhaltiger Kollagenträger (EMD 53 155 versus Sulmycin®-Implant) im Rahmen der Versorgung von Knocheninfektionen/-kontaminationen. E. Merck, Darmstadt, 1995, EMD 53 155–89.

Härle A. Infektionen. In: Bauer R, Kerschbaumer F, Poisel S (editors). Orthopädische Operationslehre. Stuttgart, New York: Georg Thieme Verlag; 1989: 451–90.

Knaepler H, Klemm K, Dingeldein E, Wahlig H. Gentamicin-PMMA-Miniketten in der septischen Knochen- und Weichteilchirurgie. Unfallchirurgie 1985; 88: 457–64.

Nies B. Prospektive randomisierte Vergleichsstudie zur Erhebung pharmakokinetischer und klinischer Daten bei Anwendung zweier gentamicinhaltiger Kollagenträger (EMD 53 155 versus Sulmycin® Implant) im Rahmen der Versorgung von Knocheninfektionen/-kontaminationen – Zwischenbericht zur Pharmakokinetik. E. Merck, Darmstadt, 1995, EMD 53 155.

QM-Arbeitsanweisung QM-AA 8511. Mikrobiologische Bestimmung der Gentamicinkonzentration in Serum und Wundsekret. E. Merck, Darmstadt, 1995, EMD 53 155–78.

QM-Arbeitsanweisung QM-AA 8512. Mikrobiologische Bestimmung der Gentamicinkonzentration im Urin. E. Merck, Darmstadt, 1995, EMD 53 155–91.

Rens van ThJG, Kayser FH (editors). Local antibiotic treatment in osteomyelitis and soft tissue infections. Excerpta Medica Amsterdam, Int. Congress Series 1981: 556.

Sachweh D. Lokale Antibiotika-Behandlung mit protrahierter Wirkstoff-Freisetzung in der Weichteilchirurgie. In: Suckert R, Vecsei V (editors). Antibiotika-Träger. Ein neuer Weg in der lokalen Infektionsbehandlung in der Chirurgie. Purkersdorf bei Wien: Medizinisch-pharmazeutische Verlagsgesellschaft, 1986: 28–32.

Suckert R, Vecsei V (editors). Antibiotika-Träger. Ein neuer Weg in der lokalen Infektionsbehandlung in der Chirurgie. Purkersdorf bei Wien: Medizinisch-pharmazeutische Verlagsgesellschaft, 1986.

Wahlig H. Gentamicin-PMMA beads, a drug delivery system; basic results. In: Van Rens ThJG, Kayser FH (Eds.). Local antibiotic treatment in osteomyelitis and soft tissue infections. Excerpta Medica Amsterdam, Int. Congress Series 1981; 556: 9–17.

Clinical Experience with a New Dual-Component Gentamicin-Collagen Fleece (Septocoll®) in the Treatment of Chronic Osteomyelitis of the Long Tubular Bones

U. Grüßner, H. Büchner, R. Göttmann

Introduction

Since the introduction of PMMA products containing gentamicin (Septopal®-chains, Septopal®-mini-chains, Merck, Darmstadt) local antibiotic therapy has become a firmly established element in the surgical treatment of bone and soft-tissue infections or contaminations (Blaha et al., 1990; Evans and Nelson, 1993; Klemm and Schnettler, 1981; Weise and Müller, 1988). In view of the successful treatment with these nonabsorbable drug carriers, endeavours were made during the last decade to develop absorbable and therefore no longer removable materials (Ascherl et al., 1989; Wernet et al., 1992). All these products, whether absorbable or not, have one aspect in common: they contain gentamicin, an antibiotic with a wide spectrum of action and many years of continued consistent resistance.

The justification for the local use of gentamicin bound to a medium arises from the requirement for efficacious antibiotic treatment at the site of infection with simultaneously slight, negligible or no systematic undesirable effects (Kloß et al., 1981). The main focus from the clinical and pharmacological points of view involves initially high local gentamicin concentrations with simultaneous protracted active ingredient release until the dermal wound healing phase (5 th to 7 th postoperative day) (Eckert, 1993). During this phase, gentamicin plasma concentrations should as far as possible not exceed the value of 2 µg/ml or if so, only for a short period, i.e. < 24 hours in order to avoid systemic undesirable effects (e.g., ototoxic or nephrotoxic effects) (Burkle, 1981; Schmidt et al., 1988; Walenkamp et al., 1986).

Gentamicin-collagen carriers possess the advantages that they adapt to the conditions of the wound as a result of their plasticity, mix with cancellous bone or bone graft material, have the possibility of cutting to size, according to the processing of the collagen, they maintain their dimensions even in a moist environment, and via the coarsely porous connection between the collagen fibers do not hinder wound healing. As a result of absorption of the collagen carrier, removal of this drug product is no longer required, so that gentamicin-collagen carriers such as the investigational preparation Septocoll® are indicated in one-step surgical procedures, surgical operations in which no "space-occupier" is required, or in surgical operations in which antibiotic coverage which goes beyond the 14-day-antibiotic therapy is not necessary. During the clinical use of such carriers, it should be observed though, that the wound is in no way "punched out", since increased secretion is possible within the context of the absorption processes.

Owing to the complexity of the clinical picture, chronic osteomyelitis requires multilayered treatment and not infrequently necessitates an individual treatment schedule which is adapted to the specific case. A *conditio sine qua non* of treatment is radical debridement of all infected and necrotic tissue, partly with repeated intervention until the infection is resolved. As an adjunctive treatment, local antibiotic carriers are increasingly being inserted into the excised wound cavity and additional systemic antibiotics administered where there is the risk or the presence of microbial colonization. Cephalosporin is used mainly here as the basic systemic antibiotic.

Local antibiotic carriers, such as the newly developed gentamicin-collagen fleece Septocoll®, have the advantage that, after excision of the infected necrotic tissue, they are inserted in the wound cavity, which is for the most part contaminated and previously damaged by surgery and prior interventions, and can therefore exert their action in the critical border zones. In the immediate vicinity of the antibiotic carrier Septocoll® gentamicin concentrations are 100 to 300 times higher than those in plasma with intravenous administration (Burkhard et al., 1981; Dingeldein, 1987, 1993; Kloß et al., 1981). The minimal inhibitory concentration (MIC) of the pathogenic bacteria is exceeded several fold with local application (Klemm and Schnettler, 1981; Walenkamp et al., 1986). Even bacteria held to be resistant could be killed off, without this being detectable locally. According to this starting point, the value of the local antibiotic carrier lies in the protection of the tissue around the excised area, i.e., in killing off residual bacteria present, in prevention of contamination of the wound by exogenous bacteria, in the prevention of bacterial colonization and a renewed flare-up of infection. Nevertheless, it is to be observed that careful debridement is indispensable and any bony sequestrum or infected portions of tissue present are to be removed. In addition, antibiotic protection exists only in the immediately adjoining layers of tissue. Therefore, with the risk or presence of bacterial colonization in the systemic circulation, additional systemic antibiotics are to be administered.

As a result of the variability of the disease (duration of disease, slight differences in the spread of infection, severity of the infection, localization of the infection, number of previous operations, time of surgery, immunological status of the patient, clinical symptoms, etc.) and the treatment options in connection with this, prospective, comparative clinical trials with the clinical picture of chronic osteomyelitis are for considerations of a biometrical (Blaha et al., 1993; Gentry and Rodriguez, 1990; Norrby, 1989), practical (Blaha et al., 1993; Widmer et al., 1988), and ethical (Blaha et al., 1993; Norrby, 1989) nature scarcely practicable or often not justifiable in the patient's interest. Particularly, a uniform, universally applicable clinical classification of the degree of severity of chronic osteomyelitis is lacking for the comparability of treatment results; an optimum treatment with validity for each patient or for a selected patient cohort likewise does not exist (Schmidt et al., 1988; Wagner et al., 1985; Widmer et al., 1988). Most clinical studies restrict themselves therefore to retrospective analyses, which reflect predominately the authors' experience with particular surgical methods or therapeutic management.

The aim of this prospective clinical study was to test the efficacy and safety of the newly developed absorbable antibiotic carrier Septocoll® in patients with chronic osteomyelitis of the long tubular bones of the upper and lower limb. The decisive period for assessment of efficacy involved the first two postoperative weeks, i.e., the period during which the drug product Septocoll®

exerts its efficacy. Independently of this, follow-up examinations to ascertain the rate of infection were performed on a compulsory basis until the 6 th postoperative week and on an optional basis until the 3 rd postoperative month.

Material and Methods

During the period from July 1992 to August 1995, 96 patients with chronic osteomyelitis of the long tubular bones of the upper and lower limb were recruited and treated with the investigational product Septocoll® in a prospective, open, uncontrolled, multicenter, multinational clinical trial. All in all, 20 trial centers from the Netherlands, Germany, France, Great Britain, and Austria took part.

Exclusively patients in whom chronic osteomyelitis had been established clinically, radiologically, chemically by laboratory analyses, and, if possible, preoperatively and bacteriologically were admitted into this prospective, open, uncontrolled clinical study. A further criterion was, with a first occurrence of the bone infection, at least 6 weeks' history of infection or the clinical picture of a recurrent bone infection. In the context of the scheduled surgical treatment, the implantation of 2 Septocoll®-fleeces – corresponding to a dose of 140 mg of gentamicin base – was prescribed as the study medication, in addition to a 7 day administration of 3×2 g of cefazolin i.v. The main study criterion was the rate of infection within the first 2 weeks after surgery. This established interval of time was regarded as the decisive period in which Septocoll® exerts its action. By fixing this interval of time, it was possible on the one hand for therapeutic follow-up operations (e.g., cancellous bone grafts) or clinically specific treatment schemes to be performed unhindered by requirements specific to the study. On the other hand, this prevented assessment of the action of Septocoll® during the first two weeks after implantation being influenced by second-look operations.

Septocoll®

The investigational drug Septocoll® (EMD 53 155) used in the present study is an absorbable collagen preparation of dimensions of 5×8 cm containing two active ingredients: firstly the tried and trusted, water-soluble and therefore rapidly available gentamicin sulfate and secondly, the newly developed hydrophobic and therefore prolonged availability gentamicin crobefate.

The collagen used in Septocoll® involves native, pure, absorbable collagen fibers obtained from the dermis of cattle hides (predominately type-I collagen), which is bound to a soft, absorbent, coarsely porous fleece. A fleece of a weight of 700 mg and dimensions of 5 × 8 cm contains a total of 70 mg of gentamicin base, including 35 mg in the form of gentamicin sulfate (58.3 mg of gentamicin sulfate) and gentamicin crobefate (179 mg of gentamicin crobefate), respectively. The collagen portion weighs approximately 463 mg.

The combination of the highly water-soluble gentamicin sulfate with the sparingly soluble, slowly dissociable gentamicin crobefate guarantees both an initially rapid and a delayed release of gentamicin, so that an action until at least the 7 th postoperative day must be assumed. Both Septocoll® fleeces were inserted once at the end of the surgical procedure, together with overflow drains, into the wound cavity before closure.

Inclusion Criteria

Patients both male and female (with contraception) of any ethnic group and over 18 years of age could be admitted into the study. The prerequisite was surgical treatment of the focus of infection in the context of an in-patient stay, in addition to the implantation of both Septocoll® fleeces (40 cm³) without surgical and technical difficulties, i.e., it must be possible to close the surgically treated wound as far as possible without tension after implantation of Septocoll® and one or several overflow drains. The additional treatment with 3 × 2 g of cefazolin over 7 days was based on the multinational nature of the study, represented the largest possible common denominator of the various methods of treatment and was selected on the basis of considerations of uniformity of the patient cohort.

Exclusion Criteria

In the context of the exclusion criteria related to the preparation, patients with known hypersensitivity to collagen/gentamicin/cefazolin, patients having received antibiotic treatment within the last two days before the scheduled operation, and patients with obvious liver damage (increase in transaminases > 2 times the normal value) or renal insufficiency (increase in serum creatinine > 1.5 mg% or creatinine clearance < 50 – 80 ml/min) were excluded.

Study Schedule

Preoperatively a detailed *case history* was obtained, including demographic data, prognostic factors (e.g., pre-existing diseases, diabetes mellitus), symptoms, accompanying diseases, and long-term medication. *Clinical examinations* were performed preoperatively and at specified times until the 6 th postoperative week (optionally until the 12 th postoperative week). Intraoperatively, it was compulsory to obtain *bacteriological* samples: for this, 1 swabbing from the infected soft tissue and the infected bone cavity and/or one bone and soft-tissue biopsy, respectively, were to be taken. After isolation and differentiation of the pathogens, an antibiotic sensitivity test was to be performed at least for gentamicin and cefazolin. In addition, bacteriological material for examination was to be obtained both preoperatively if a fistula was present or in the context of a diagnostic puncture and postoperatively in the event of renewed infection. *X-ray examinations* were scheduled preoperatively, on postoperative days 0 – 8 and 12 – 16, in addition to after 12 weeks. The *laboratory examinations* performed at the same times included the following parameters: total blood count, including differential blood count, ESR, C-reactive protein, LDH, SGOT, γ-GT, alkaline phosphatase, total bilirubin, total protein, glucose, retentional and essential electrolyte values. In addition, urine samples were taken to determine the pH value, haemoglobin, protein and glucose, in addition to urinary sedimentation.

Surgical Therapy

Surgical therapy comprised one-step surgical treatment of the focus of infection, with removal of bony sequestra or non-vital portions of bone, in addition to infected and necrotic bone and soft tissue. Repeated intervention with the performance of second-look operations was not scheduled, for considerations relating to the assessment of efficacy of the investigational drug Septocoll®. Likewise, the use of antibiotic rinsing solutions or local antibiotic carrier other than Septocoll® was not allowed. Primary closure of the wound was imperatively specified.

Results

All 96 patients admitted into the study with the diagnosis of chronic osteomyelitis received the prescribed implantation of a dose of 2 Septocoll® fleeces (140 mg of gentamicin base) in the context of the surgical measure before closure of the wound. Accompanying treatment with 3 × 2 g of cefazolin i.v. was administered correctly in 87 patients. In 9 of the 96 patients (9.4%), irregularities occurred in the accompanying antibiotic treatment, either in that no treatment, shorter treatment or longer treatment with cefazolin was administered, or that other antibiotics were administered. Since no decisive influence on the results was observed as a consequence thereof, these patients were included in the assessment.

Of the 96 patients admitted into the study, 26 were female and 70 patients were male. Almost ¾ of the patients, therefore, were men. The average age over both sexes was 47 ± 18 years, with a minimum of 19 and a maximum of 87 years (Table **1**).

In 73 patients (Table **2**), the chronic osteomyelitis occurred after fractures. In 32 cases, closed fractures were involved and in 41 cases, open fractures. The open fractures were of the first degree in 8 cases, second degree in 16 cases, and third degree in 14 cases. A further 3 patients presented with open fractures without information on severity.

In an additional 14 of the 96 patients, postoperative osteomyelitis was involved. In 3 patients, this involved haematogenic osteomyelitis and in 2 patients iatrogenic osteomyelitis which occurred after intra-articular injection. In one case, chronic osteomyelitis was the result of a pressure sore, one a burn, and one bursitis with superinfection. In one case, information on the cause was lacking.

Table **1** Demographic characteristics

Parameter	Men	Total cohort Women	Total
Number of patients	70	26	96
Age (years)	45 ± 18	52 ± 17	47 ± 18
[min – max]	19 – 87	22 – 57	19 – 87
Height (cm)*	177 ± 7	165 ± 7	173 ± 9
Weight (kg)*	80 ± 17	72 ± 15	76 ± 17

* missing data of 3 patients

Table **2** Cause of chronic osteomyelitis

Cause of chronic osteomyelitis	Number of patients/ Percentage distribution	
Fractures	73	(76.0%)
Closed fractures	32	
Open fractures	41	
1st deg. open fractures	8	
2nd deg. open fractures	16	
3rd deg. open fractures	14	
Open fractures with no information on degree	3	
Postoperative osteomyelitis	14	(14.6%)
Haematogenic osteomyelitis	3	(3.1%)
Post-intra-articular injection	2	(2.1%)
Burn	1	(1.0%)
Pressure sore	1	(1.0%)
Bursitis	1	(1.0%)
Missing data	1	

In 89 patients, more specific information on the interval between occurrence of injury and the scheduled operation could be obtained (Table **3**). Only in 7 cases did injury date from 4–12 weeks. In 20 patients a history of osteomyelitis of 3–12 weeks was present. In 29 patients (32.6% of the patients, respectively), the time of injury was 1–5 years, in 30 patients (or 33.7% of cases) 6–60 years previously. In almost $^2/_3$ of the cases, chronic osteomyelitis had existed therefore for longer than one year.

Table **3**   Duration of the disease

Interval between trauma and actual operation

Time interval (weeks, year)	No. of patients
1– 4 weeks	n = 1
4– 8 weeks	n = 4
8–12 weeks	n = 2
12–26 weeks	n = 10
27–52 weeks	n = 10
1– 5 years	n = 29
6–10 years	n = 8
11–60 years	n = 22

Except for 5 patients and one patient without more precise information, the remaining 90 patients had for the most part undergone repeated surgery. In detail, the distribution of previous surgery was as follows (Table **4**): 50% of the patients (n = 48) had undergone 1–3 previous operations and 43.75% of the patients (n = 42) more than 3 previous operations. In one patient, 33 previous operations had been performed before the scheduled surgery.

Table **4**   Previous operations

Previous operation	
No. of operations	No. of patients
None	n = 5
1 pre-op	n = 8
2 pre-op	n = 18
3 pre-op	n = 22
4 pre-op	n = 12
5 pre-op	n = 10
6–10 pre-op	n = 13
11–15 pre-op	n = 6
33 pre-op	n = 1
Missing data	n = 1

Clinical symptoms were observed preoperatively in 94 patients (97.9%). In addition to erythema, swelling, hyperthermia, pain and/or functional impairment, in 62 patients (64.6%) fistulas, in 20 patients (20.8%) an abscess and in 7 patients (7.3%) a phlegmon were present. In 52 patients (54.2%) suppuration was documented.

Chronic osteomyelitis was located on the lower limb in 87.5% (n = 84) of the patients included and on the upper limb in only 12.5% (n = 12) of cases (Fig.**1**). The site of predilection on the lower limb was the tibia (and fibula) with 51% (n = 49); in 36.5% (n = 35) of cases, the femur was affected. In the upper limb, osteomyelitis occurred most frequently on the humerus (n = 10; 10.4%). There were no significant differences in the distribution of localization according to right or left limbs for the corresponding bone sections. Therefore, in 52.1% of all cases (n = 50) the right

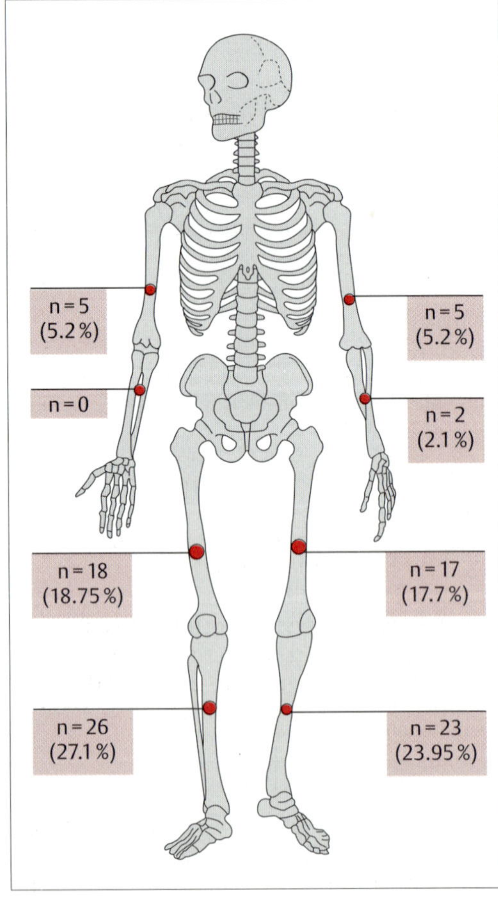

Fig.**1**   Site of manifestation of chronic osteomyelitis.

half of the body was involved and in 47.9% (n = 46) the left half.

The extraction of biopsies and/or swabbings from the site of infection was scheduled intra-operatively. In 74 cases (77.1% of the cases respectively) a bone biopsy was performed and in 82 cases (85.4% of cases) a bone swabbing was carried out. In 91 of the 96 patients (94.8%) therefore, either a bone biopsy or a bone swabbing was performed intraoperatively.

The taking of soft-tissue biopsies and soft-tissue swabbings was formed in 66 and 75 patients (with 68.75% and 78.13% respectively). In 82 of the 96 cases (85.4%) either a soft-tissue biopsy or a soft-tissue swabbing was performed.

Over the entire patient cohort, the intra-operative result of either a bone or soft tissue biopsy, or a bone or soft tissue swabbing existed for 93 patients (96.8%). Only in 3 patients (3.1%) was no material for examination obtained intra-operatively. In 1 of these 3 patients, a preoperative bacteriological finding (puncture fluid) was available.

In 52 of the 96 patients, taking into account all the intraoperative biopsies and swabbings, monoinfections were involved and in 15 patients, mixed infections. In 26 cases, the material for examination obtained intraoperatively was sterile, even though the preoperative samples in a further 8 cases yielded a positive bacteriological finding. With respect to the mixed infections, up to 4 different bacteria occurred in the patients (Table **5**).

The bacterial spectrum collected shows clearly the prime significance of *Staphylococcus aureus* and *Staphylococcus epidermidis,* which it was possible to detect in 74.6% (n = 50 of 67) and 11.9% (n = 8 of 67) of all positive samples (Table **6**). In 14 cases, gentamicin-resistant and in 4 cases gentamicin-moderately sensitive pathogens occurred either as single pathogens or together with gentamicin-sensitive pathogens.

In 8 of the 96 patients (8.3%), infections occurred within the first 14 postoperative days. In 3 of these 8 patients, the site of implantation of Septocoll was not identical to the site of the postoperative infection: insertion of the Septocoll®

fleeces was periosteal or osteal; the infection occurred, however, subcutaneously.

In 5 of the 8 cases (5.2%) a postoperative infection occurred in which the site of implantation for Septocoll® was identical to that of the infection. In 2 of these cases, gentamicin-resistant bacteria could be distinguished in the intraoperatively obtained material for bacteriological examination and in one further case, foreign matter (TEP) was left in the site of infection. Among these 5 infections, 2 deep infections were involved and 3 cases of combined superficial and deep infection.

In 2 of the 8 cases, it was necessary to perform a revision operation for treatment of the infection. The remaining infections healed under conservative therapeutic measures.

Healing progressed in 75.6% (n = 68 of 90) of the patients until the 14 th postoperative day primarily and in 24.4% of the patients secondarily. In 13 patients (14.4%) a haematoma occurred during postoperative evolution which emptied spontaneously in 9 cases, was punctured in 2 cases, or resorbed in 2 cases. In 20 patients (22.2%), a seroma was observed, which emptied spontaneously in 15 cases, was punctured in 2 cases, and resolved spontaneously in 3 cases. The punctured seromas were sterile in both cases.

Possible or probable adverse events related to the use of Septocoll® were rare. By way of severe adverse events, in addition to the revision operations and operations for further treatment of the patients (e.g., cancellous bone grafts), firstly severe bleeding after TEP explantation with subsequent revision on the same day and secondly a death as a result of a cardiac and circulatory failure in tumoral disease occurred.

Discussion

Treatment of chronic osteomyelitis is fundamentally surgical, with surgical removal of all sequestered, non-vital necrotic and infected bone and soft tissue. Therapy consists as a rule of multiple-stage intervention, encompassing primarily treatment of infection, secondarily reduction of

Table **5**   Number of pathogens

	Pathogen 1	Pathogen 2	Pathogen 3	Pathogen 4
Number of patients	52	10	3	2

Bacteriological spectrum*	No. of patients			Table **6** Bacterial spectrum
	Mono-infections	Mixed infections	Total	
Gram-positive pathogens				
Staphylococcus aureus	40	10	50	
Staphylococcus epidermis	4	4	8	
Staphylococcus lugdunensis	1	–	1	
Coag. neg. *Staphylococcus* w.f.i.**	1	–	1	
β-haemolytic *Streptococci* of the B group	–	2	2	
Streptococcus agalactiae	–	1	1	
Streptococcus faecalis	–	1	1	
Enterococcus	1	–	1	
Enterococcus specificus	–	2	2	
Enterococcus faecalis	–	1	1	
Cocci	–	1	1	
Corynebacterium species	–	2	2	
Gram-negative phatogens				
Pseudomonas aeruginosa	3	2	5	
Proteus species	1	–	1	
Proteus mirabilis	–	1	1	
E. coli	–	3	3	
Enterobacter cloacae	1	1	2	
Citrobacter diversus	–	2	2	
Lactobacillus	–	1	1	
Anaerobes w.f.i.	–	2	2	
Bacteroides	–	1	1	
Total	**52**	**37**	**88**	

*   Multiple mentions per patient possible.
** Without further information.

the bone defect, and thirdly removal of the bone defect (Wittek et al., 1988).

Without exception, patients with florid infection and scheduled treatment of infection were included in the present study, in whom the collagen carrier containing gentamicin, Septocoll® was used as adjunctive local antibiotic treatment. In the context of this study, it was deliberately refrained from recourse to second-look operations. Directly opposed to the advantage of second-look operations, the new cleansing and refreshing of the wound, is an additional burden on the patient as a result of a second operation. We were of the opinion that effective primary surgery and additional administration of the local antibiotic carrier Septocoll® ought to be sufficient for the treatment of infection. In addition, it appeared to us not to be justified in the context of the study protocol to prescribe second-look operations generally for all patients, all the more since the decision for such an operation is taken rather more individually and is not the rule in all the participating countries. The rate of infection of 5.2% recorded during the first 14 postoperative days appears to corroborate this opinion.

The use of Septocoll® as adjunctive therapy in the treatment of osteomyelitis can be supported without restriction on the basis of the success rate of 94.8%. The low rate of infection refers though purely to the first postoperative days, i.e., to the period during which Septocoll® exerts its activity. A longer observation time appears admittedly to be desirable from a clinical point of view in the clinical picture of chronic osteomyelitis. For a consideration of the efficacy of a local antibiotic carrier, the period of action of the local drug product is, however, decisive.

The method of action of local antibiotic carrier should once again become clear from the following discussion. Since this applies to all local antibiotic carriers, reference is to be made only in passing to the present study.

In considering the efficacy of a local antibiotic carrier, it should be distinguished in which tissues the drug carrier is to be implanted and in which layers of tissue the postoperative infection occurs: in principle, the activity of a local antibiotic carrier exists only at the respective site of implantation and in the immediately adjoining layers of tissue. In periosteal or osteal implantation of the antibiotic carrier, protection of the subcutaneous tissue does not inevitably exist, above all not when the tissue layers are separated from one another by closure of the fascia. The superficial, i.e., subcutaneous infections observed in 3 patients in the present study result from subcutaneous bacterial foci left behind, into which the antibiotic could not diffuse due to the chosen site of implantation. This does not imply that the method of action of the locally applied antibiotic carrier must be called into question, but rather that natural limits are imposed here on the antibiotic carrier. A further factor is the necessarily radical nature of the surgery, which is not to be replaced even by the implantation of an antibiotic carrier. With a follow-up operation within 2 days owing to persistent infection, it is highly probable to assume an excessively tissue-sparing surgical procedure.

Today, it continues to be assumed that the sensitivity or the resistance of a pathogen represents an absolute characteristic, which in the event of resistance leads at least in the majority of cases – if not inevitably – to a persistent infection. According to Grimm, categorization into sensitive, moderately sensitive, and resistant applies only for systemic antibiotics and not for local antibiotic treatment with its far higher gentamicin concentrations (Grimm, 1989; Rodloff, 1988). This is confirmed in correlation with clinical medicine on the basis of the bacterial spectrum obtained in the present study. Of 17 of the patients included in the study with gentamicin-resistant or moderately sensitive bacteria, either in mono or mixed culture, only 2 patients presented with a persistent infection. This means that only every 8th patient with resistant or moderately sensitive bacteria under treatment with Septocoll® within the first 14 postoperative days showed an infection. Even if a globalized rate for local antibiotic therapy under conditions of resistant bacteria is not possible in view of the low number of cases, these results should be an occasion for extensive tests.

Via the 7 day application of cephazolin, the question naturally arises as to which of the two antibiotics, the locally implanted Septocoll® or the parenterally administered cefazolin, is responsible for which action. Basically, it is considered that the action of systemically administered antibiotics in relation to the site of surgery is limited in the immediate postoperative phase, since as a result of surgery (i.e., by excision of tissue, blockage of vessels by ligation or electrocautery, inserted hooks or clamps) swelling of tissue and consequently micro- and macrocirculatory disturbances occur (Burkhard et al., 1981). It is extremely difficult to supply proof of the valency of one or other of the antibiotics. Nevertheless 14 patients with cefazolin resistant or moderately sensitive bacteria were included in the present study. Only in 2 cases did an infection occur in the first 14 postoperative days, one of which involved a patient with both cefazolin and also gentamicin resistant bacteria. If one assumes that, at least in the patient with cefazolin resistant bacteria, cefazolin can achieve no adequate effect, freedom from infection is to be ascribed to the surgical operation and to Septocoll®.

With respect to localization and pathogen distribution, there were no strong differences between the literature (Weise and Müller, 1988) and the data collected in the study. The site of predilection for chronic osteomyelitis is the tibia. The most frequent bacteria are *Staphylococcus aureus* and *Staphylococcus epidermidis* pathogens.

The high haematoma and seroma rate of 14.4 and 22.2%, respectively, recorded in the study within the first 14 days can be attributed partially to the effects of the study. In 92 patients, implantation of both Septocoll® fleeces was osteal, periosteal, or subfascial, so that a correlation with the implanted Septocoll® is very unlikely. Only in 4 patients was 1 Septocoll® fleece respectively inserted subcutaneously. A haematoma was observed in none of these patients. In one of these 4 patients though, a seroma emptied spontaneously within the first 7 postoperative days. The conspiciously high seroma rate could possibly be attributed to a disproportion between the size of the wound and the strict instructions to implant 2 Septocoll® fleeces. In wider use, this ought to be avoided by a wound-sized dose adaptation.

Severe adverse events due to the preparation did not occur. In none of the 96 patients was it necessary to remove Septocoll® due to adverse events.

Conclusion

In clinical use in bone and soft-tissue infections, the following conclusions may be drawn from the experience gained to date with Septocoll®:
1. Reliable efficacy within the first 2 weeks.
2. High local antibiotic concentrations within the first 7 postoperative days.
3. Good tissular safety.
4. Low risk of sensitization.
5. Low tendency of development of resistance.
6. Good handling properties.

References

Ascherl R, Stemberger A, Geißdörfer K, Claudi B, Machka K, Lechner F, Blümel G. Experimentelle Ergebnisse und erste klinische Erfahrungen mit Kollagen-Gentamicin als Zusatzmaßnahme bei der chronischen Osteomyelitis. In: Stemberger A, Ascherl R, Lechner F, Blümel G (eds.). Kollagen als Wirkstoffträger – Einsatzmöglichkeiten in der Chirurgie. Stuttgart, New York: Schattauer, 1989: 45–53.

Blaha JD, Nelson CL, Frevert LF, Henry SL, Seligson DK, Esterhai JL, Heppenstall RB, Calhoun J, Cobos J, Mader J. The use of Septopal (polymethylmethacrylate beads with gentamicin) in the treatment of chronic osteomyelitis. Istr Course Lect 1990; 39: 509.

Blaha JD, Calhoun JH, Nelson CL et al. Comparison of the clinical efficacy and tolerance of Gentamicin-PMMA beads on surgical wire versus combined and systemic therapy for osteomyelitis. Clin Orthop 1993; 295: 8–12.

Burkhard K, Kloß H-P, Grüßner U. Pharmakokinetik eines neuen Gentamicin-Kollagen-Vlieses (EMD 53155). In: Schultheis K-H, Rehm KE, Ecke H (eds.). Chirurgische Infektionen von Knochen, Gelenken und Weichteilen. Berlin, New York: Walter De Gruyter, 1981: 69–78.

Burkle WS. Comparative evaluation of the aminoglycoside antibiotics for systemic use. Drug Intelligence and Clinical Pharmacy 1981; 15: 847–62.

Dingeldein E. EMD 53155 – Gentamicin-Kollagenvlies: Untersuchungen zur Gentamicinfreisetzung *in vitro*. E. Merck, Darmstadt, 1987, EMD 53155–112.

Dingeldein E. EMD 53155 – Gentamicinkonzentration in Körperflüssigkeiten von Patienten nach Implantation von Gentamicin-Kollagenvlies in Verbindung mit einer Redondrainage. E. Merck, Darmstadt, 1993, EMD 53155–167.

Eckert P. Gentamycin-Kollagen in der Behandlung infizierter Knochen und Weichteilschäden. In: Gahr RH (ed.). Entwicklungen in der Unfallchirurgie, Rückblick-Ausblick. Springer-Verlag, Berlin, Heidelberg, New York; 1993: 214–8.

Evans RP, Nelson CL. Gentamicin-impregnated polymethylmethacrylate beads compared with systemic antibiotic therapy in the treatment of chronic osteomyelitis. Clinical Orthopaedics and Related Research 1993; 295: 37–42.

Gentry LO, Rodriguez GG. Oral ciprofloxacin compared with parenteral antibiotics in the treatment of osteomyelitis. Antimicrob Agents Chemother 1990; 34: 40–3.

Grimm H. Bakteriologische und pharmakokinetische Aspekte der topischen Antibiotikaanwendung. In: Stemberger A, Ascherl R, Lechner F, Blümel G (eds.). Kollagen als Wirkstoffträger – Einsatzmöglichkeiten in der Chirurgie. Stuttgart, New York: Schattauer, 1989: 33–7.

Klemm K, Schnettler R. Gentamicin-PMMA-Ketten. In: Schultheis K-H, Rehm KE, Ecke H (eds.). Chirurgische Infektionen von Knochen, Gelenken und Weichteilen. Berlin, New York: Walter De Gruyter, 1981: 45–57.

Kloß H-P, Burkhard K, Grüßner U. Erste klinische Ergebnisse mit einem neuen Gentamicin-Kollagen-Vlies (EMD 53155). In: Schultheis K-H, Rehm KE, Ecke H (eds.). Chirurgische Infektionen von Knochen, Gelenken und Weichteilen. Berlin, New York: Walter De Gruyter, 1981: 59–68.

Norrby SR. Ciprofloxacin in the treatment of acute and chronic osteomyelitis: a review. Scand J Infect Dis 1989; 60 (Suppl): 74–8.

Rodloff AC. Antibiotische Therapie bei Wund- und Knocheninfektionen. In: Schmidt HGK (ed.). Knochen- und Weichteilinfektionen 1988: 33–7.

Schmidt HGK, Neikes M, Wittek F. Chirurgische Systematik von akuten und chronischen Knocheninfektionen. In: Schmidt HGK (ed.). Knochen- und Weichteilinfektionen 1988: 67–72.

Stahlmann R, Lode H. Welche Faktoren erhöhen die Nephrotoxizität von Aminoglykosid-Antibiotika? Dt med Wschr 1986; 111: 1409–14.

Wagner DK, Collier BD, Rytel MW. Long-term intravenous antibiotic therapy in chronic osteomyelitis. Arch Intern Med 1985; 145: 1073–8.

Walenkamp GHIM, Vree TB, Van Rens TJG. Gentamicin-PMMA beads – pharmacokinetic and nephrotoxicological study. Clinical Orthopaedics 1986; 205: 171–83.

Weise K, Müller HP. Die lokale Antibiotikatherapie bei postoperativer und posttraumatischer Osteitis mit der Septopal®-Kette. Unfallchirurg 1988; 91: 416–21.

Wernet E, Ekkernkamp A, Jellestad H, Muhr G. Antibiotikahaltiges Kollagenvlies in der Osteitistherapie. Unfallchirurg 1992; 95: 259–64.

Widmer A, Barraud GE, Zimmerli W. Reaktivierung einer *Staphylococcus-aureus*-Osteomyelitis nach 49 Jahren. Schweiz med Wschr 1988; 118: 23–6.

Wittek F, Schmidt HGK, Neikes M. Therapie der chronischen Knocheninfektion. In: Schmidt HGK (ed). Knochen- und Weichteilinfektionen 1988: 73–82.

2

The Biomaterial PMMA

Physical and Chemical Properties of Bone Cements

W. Ege, K.-D. Kühn, C. Tuchscherer, H. Maurer

Introduction

All bone cements on the market today are based on methyl methacrylate (density: $0.95\,g/cm^3$; boiling point: $100\,°C$; molecular weight: 100.0).

$$CH_3$$
$$H_2C=C-C-OCH_3$$
$$O$$

Methyl methacrylate

The $C=C$ double bonding allows the polymerization of the molecule. To start the polymerization process we need catalysts. One is benzoyl peroxide.

Benzoyl peroxide (BPO)

BPO is a white crystalline mass stabilized by means of about 25% of water to prevent explosion. The BPO is mixed into the powder.

To start the reaction at room temperature a so-called cocatalyst is needed, the dimethyl-p-toluidine. It is a liquid and is dissolved in the monomer in the ampoule.

N,N-dimethyl-*p*-toluidine (DMPT)

At the moment when powder and monomer are mixed together benzoyl radicals are formed.

$$DMPT + BPO \longrightarrow \quad (= R\cdot)$$

These radicals $\mathbf{R}\cdot$ now start the polymerization by breaking up the $C-C$ double bonding.

growth of polymer chains

As there is a large number of radicals a large number of chains is formed. These chains are linear and not cross-linked.

The process is very sensitive to temperature. At lower ambient temperature it is slow, but much faster at high room temperature. Besides the temperature, the relative humidity influences the polymerization process. Below 45% r. h. the process is delayed for about 2 to 3 minutes.

During the polymerization process, energy, in the form of heat, is generated. Tests according to the ISO standard result in peak temperatures of up to $80\,°C$. *In vivo* (in the human body) only temperatures between 40 and $50\,°C$ have been measured (Biel et al., 1974).

A radical polymerization never reaches 100% conversion. Immediately after the end of the reaction about 3 to 5% of residual monomer can be detected. When stored in saline solution at $37\,°C$ the residual monomer content of test specimens drops to about 0.5% because of the slowly ongoing reaction. Only 0.5% of the monomer is released from the bone cement surface during the first days (Rudigier et al., 1991).

Mechanical Properties of Bone Cements

The following Tables **1** and **2** show some quasi-static results of different bone cements.

The addition of antibiotics influences the mechanical strength. An absolute disaster, however, is the mixing of antibiotics dissolved in water. Since water is not miscible, either with the monomer or with the polymer, a totally inhomogeneous mixture is the result (Lautenschlager et al., 1976). Table **2** shows the dramatic influence.

Therefore a serious warning against adding liquid antibiotics to bone cement is indicated.

The conclusion of the static tests is that the various bone cements do not differ very much, which, by reason of their composition, is not surprising.

In the late seventies another test was introduced, the so-called fatigue test. In this test specimens are treated with different loads at a frequency of about 5 Hz to the breaking point.

Plitz et al. (1987) and Mittelmeier et al. (1987) compared different bone cements as to their fatigue behavior. Both methods used are quite different but one can see that cements with higher quasi-static values are not in the same range after fatigue testing. However, both methods show that low viscosity bone cements are weaker than standard viscosity bone cements (Figs. **1** and **2**).

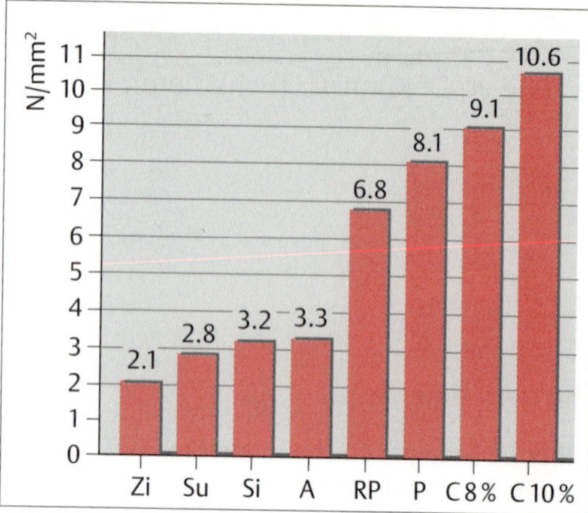

Fig. 1   Strength of various bone cements (after Hopf et al., Med. Orthop. Techn. 1985; 105: 20–5). A: Acrybond; Si: Simplex; Su: Sulfix®-6; Zi: Zimmer bone cement.

Soltesz (1993) has modified the 4-point bending test, according to ISO 5833, to a fatigue test. In this test the specimens are saturated with water at 37 °C and the tests are run in Ringer's solution at 37 °C. Variations of one bone cement (different mixing parameters) are compared.

Table **1**   Properties of bone cements

Bone cement	Compressive strength MPa (ISO)	Bending strength MPa (Dynstat)	Impact strength kJ/m² (Dynstat)
Palacos R	96	85	4.7
Palacos R + Gentamicin	95	71	3.0
Osteopal	112	98	5.0
Cement 1	100	74	3.2
Cement 2	110	95	4.8
Cement 3	89	81	2.6
Cement 4	84	70	2.0
Cement 5	78	71	2.6
Cement 6	93	75	2.0

Table **2**   Bone cements and aqueous antibiotics

Bone cement	Added gentamicin (in aqueous solution)	Compressive strength MPa
Simplex P	0	ca. 85
Simplex P	0.5 g/40 g powder	ca. 62
Palacos R	0	ca. 98
Palacos R	0.5 g/40 g powder	ca. 55

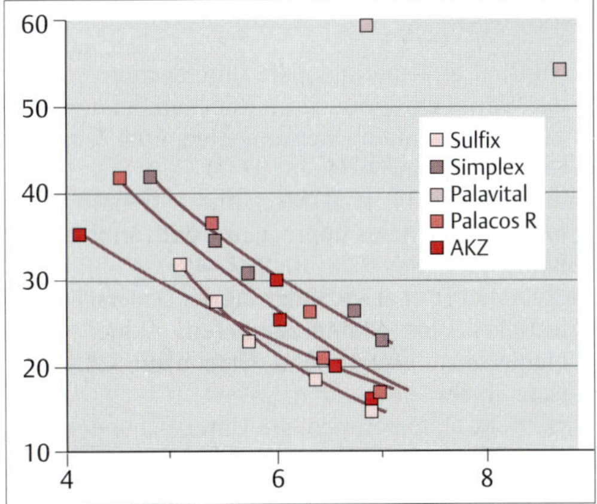

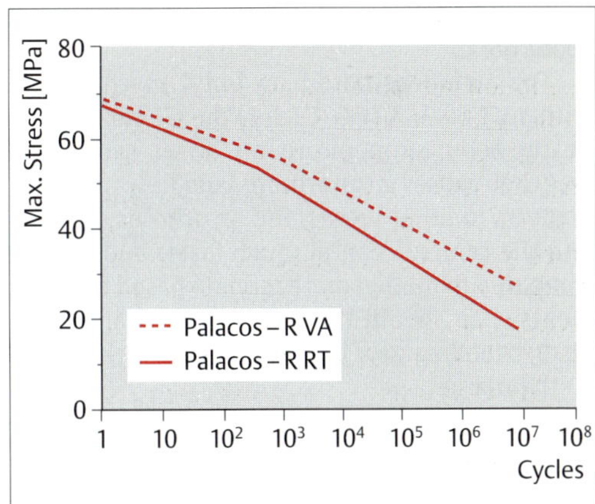

Fig. **2** Strength of various bone cements (after Plitz et al., 1987).

Fig. **3** Comparison of the stress/cycle curves of conventionally and vacuum-mixed specimens.

Two sets of specimens were prepared. For reference, the material was mixed by hand at room temperature, as well known. The second set was made by mixing the chilled powder and liquid (about 4 °C) in vacuum (about 200 mbar). The results are shown in Figure 3.

Whereas the quasi-static values do not differ significantly (67.6 and 69.0 MPa, respectively) it is obvious that the materials are weakened with increasing cycle number. After 10^7 cycles (corresponding to about 3 to 5 years of walking) only 26 % (17.8 MPa) of the initial strength of the conventionally prepared material remain, but 40 % (27.3 MPa) of the vacuum-mixed. In other words: at a given load level the vacuum-mixed specimens "survive" about ten times longer.

Some years ago, the glass transition temperature (GT) of bone cements came into discussion.

New bone cements using higher methacrylates (such as butyl methacrylate) instead of methyl methacrylate were stated to have advantageously lower GTs compared to the conventional ones. It was said that, for instance, Simplex P or Palacos had a GT of about 100 °C. In order to understand the significance of GT one must consider that if you heat up a bone cement specimen it will expand linearly as all materials do. At a distinct temperature, which varies for different polymers, the polymer chains start moving and linear elongation is no longer observed. On further heating the specimens change to a soft state.

When we determined the GT of different bone cements, we found that water-saturated specimens had a GT of about 15 to 20 °C lower than dry samples (Table **3**). For example, the GT of a dry cement specimen was about 85 °C whereas

Table **3** Glass transition temperature (°C) of bone cements

Storage Time	24 hours	2 weeks	4 weeks	24 hours	1 week	2 weeks	4 weeks	8 weeks
Storage Condition	dry 37 °C			in water 37 °C				
Palacos R	90.0	86.0	86.0	79.0	78.0	66.0	67.0	67.0
Palacos R with Gentamicin	82.0	84.0	86.0	74.0	76.0	67.0	66.0	65.0
Osteopal	94.0	92.0	93.0	92.0	85.0	84.0	68.0	70.0
Osteopal with Gentamicin	92.0	88.0	92.0	92.0	82.0	73.0	68.0	68.0
CMW1 with Gentamicin	76.0	82.0	78.0	67.0	77.0	77.0	68.0	69.0
CMW3 with Gentamicin	87.0	90.0	93.0	88.0	86.0	80.0	68.0	67.0
Palavit LV	92.0	89.0	90.0	88.0	84.0	81.0	69.0	69.0
Palavit HV	88.0	86.0	87.0	91.0	85.0	81.0	68.0	70.0
Simplex P	100.0	87.0	89.0	74.0	89.0	85.0	70.0	72.0

the same cement, water-saturated, softened at about 65 °C.

For a cement based on butyl methacrylate with a GT of about 50 °C (dry) the GT can drop to nearly body temperature on water saturation. This then causes an enormous cold flow in the cement or, in other words, the prostheses can sink into the cement mantel much faster and further compared to methyl methacrylate based bone cements. One should thus be very critical of promising-looking new bone cements which appear on the market.

References

Biehl G, et al. Experimentelle Untersuchungen über die Wärmeentwicklung im Knochen bei der Polymerisation von Knochenzementen. Arch. f. orthop. Unfall-Chirurgie 1974; 78: 62–9.

Lautenschlager EP, et al. Mechanical strength of acrylic bone cements impregnated with antibiotics. J Biomed Mat Res 1976; 10: 837–45.

Mittelmeier H, et al. Veränderung der Dauerschwingfestigkeit von PMMA-Zementen. Aktuelle Probleme in Chirurgie und Orthopädie 31. Verlag Hans Huber 1987.

Plitz W, et al. Experimentelle Untersuchungen zum Dauerschwingverhalten von Knochenzementen. Aktuelle Probleme in Chirurgie und Orthopädie 31. Verlag Hans Huber 1987.

Rudigier J, et al. Restmonomerabnahme und -freisetzung aus Knochenzementen. Untersuchungen an Laborproben und im Tierexperiment. Unfallchirurgie 1991; 7: 132–7.

Soltesz U, et al. Influence of mixing conditions on the fatigue behaviour of an acrylic bone cement. Presented at the European Biomaterials Congress, Davos 1993.

Comparison of Different Bone Cements: An Overview

Å. S. Carlsson

In this overview I intend to make comparisons of different bone cements from the clinician's point of view and present observations that are or may be of importance for the longevity of joint implants, notably total hip prostheses.

A substantial number of publications have demonstrated improved clinical and radiographic results using modern cementing techniques (Roberts et al., 1986; Russotti et al., 1988; Mulroy and Harris, 1990; Barrack et al., 1992; Östen et al., 1994). The so-called third generation technique implies that the femoral canal is thoroughly cleaned by mechanical means including high pressure lavage and occluded distally by a plug. Thereafter the canal is filled with bone cement, either mixed in vacuum or centrifuged, in a retrograde fashion from a cement gun. The cement is compressed until it reaches a doughy stage which is the time to introduce the stem prosthesis. The reamed acetabulum is correspondingly cleaned and the cement compressed until introducing the acetabular component. In a matched pair cohort study of 402 Charnley hips, Önsten et al. (1994) demonstrated a significantly increased 7-year radiographic survival of stems implanted with this third generation cementing technique compared to those implanted with Charnley's original technique. For the acetabular components the survival was significantly increased in rheumatic patients whereas the survival in osteoarthrosis was already very high even with the original technique.

Regarding the various bone cements as such, very little is to be learned from the literature and the reasons will be discussed below. Information on low vs. high viscosity cements based on methyl methacrylate (MMA) can only be found in one controlled clinical trial, in one radiostereometric (RSA) study, and in two national registers.

The interest in cements of low viscosity began with the investigations performed by Joe Miller and his group in Montreal and who demonstrated the superiority of such cements in penetrating into cancellous bone. It was assumed that the stability of an implant thereby should be improved (Miller et al., 1979). Also, Noble and Swartz (1983) injected bone cements of different viscosity into standardized pieces of cancellous bone and demonstrated that cements of low viscosity penetrated significantly deeper. In 1993 Carlsson et al. published the results of a randomized multicenter study comparing the standard viscosity cements Palacos R and Refobacin Palacos R with the low viscosity cements EMD 42 521 and EMD 42 522 supplied by the E. Merck Company, Darmstadt. With very slight modifications the low viscosity cements are now marketed as Osteopal and Osteopal G, respectively. No difference in survival or in the rate of radiographic loosening of either component was observed. Unfortunately, the power of this study was only 50 per cent, but if there had been a 10 per cent difference between the cement brands this difference should have been revealed.

Radiostereometry (RSA) – a precise method for evaluation of micromotion – was used by Mjöberg et al. (1990) for comparing 8 Scan hip prostheses fixed with Refobacin Palacos R and 8 Scan hip prostheses fixed with Palacos E-flow with gentamicin, the latter being the same brand as Osteopal G. Four acetabular components in each group migrated cranially and three femoral components in the low viscosity group and one in the high viscosity migrated distally. The authors conclude that low viscosity cement does not provide improved prosthetic fixation (Fig. 1).

The Norwegian Arthroplasty Register has supplied orthopedic surgeons with important information, not only regarding various implant designs, but also regarding types of bone cement (Havelin et al., 1995). Of the various high viscosity cement brands, CMW 1, Palacos R, Refobacin Palacos R, and Simplex had been used in a sufficient number of cases to allow an analysis and of the low viscosity cements only CMW 3. In addition a chemically different, new bone cement,

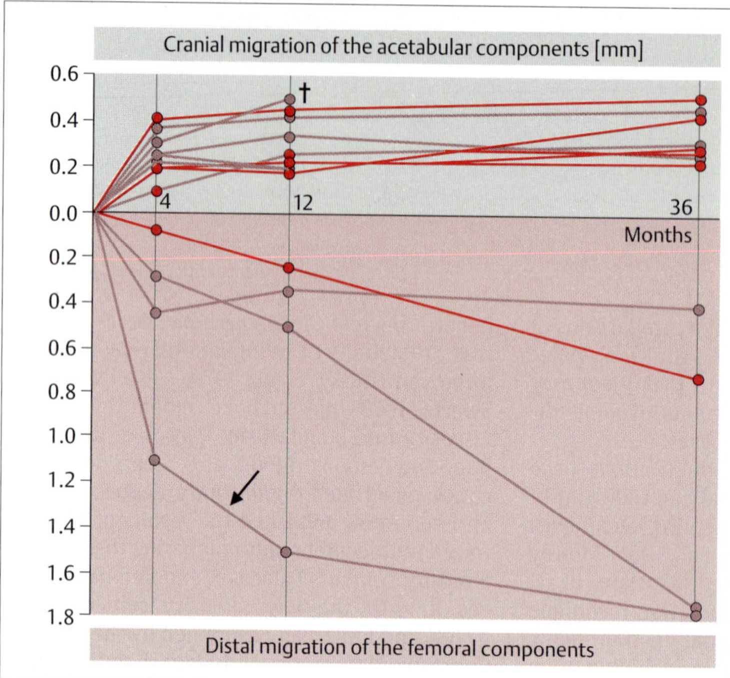

Fig. 1 Migration along the longitudinal axis of the migrating eight acetabular and four femoral components. (Eight acetabular and 10 femoral components did not migrate during the observation period.) ● = low-viscosity (Palacos E cum gentamicin, Merck) and ● = high-viscosity cement (Palacos R cum gentamicin, Merck). Arrow indicates the femoral component associated with slight pain initially at weightbearing. Palacos E cum gentamicin = Osteopal G. (from Mjöberg et al., Acta Orthopaedica Scandinavica 1990; 61: 273–4, with the permission of the author and Acta Orthopaedica Scandinavica).

Boneloc, could be evaluated. There was no difference in survival of hips implanted with the use of either of the high viscosity cements and the estimated survival rate for this group of cements of up to seven years was significantly better than for hips fixated with low viscosity cement (Fig. 2). The lowest survival rate was observed for the newly introduced and differently based Boneloc. The behavior of this cement brand will be discussed further below. Similar results with respect to MMA-based high and low viscosity bone cements have been observed in the Swedish National Hip Register (unpublished data).

LVC (Zimmer) is another MMA based bone cement of low viscosity and which has been widely used in the USA. In laboratory tests, Davies et al. (1989) found the fatigue life of this cement to be low. The clinical inferiority was revealed in a report by Granhed et al. (1991). From 1981 to 1984, 532 Charnley hips were implanted in Gothenburg and Karlstad, Sweden. After 7 – 9 years, 20 per cent of these hips had been revised and another 15 per cent were radiographically loose. Surprisingly, this is, to my knowledge, the only report on the clinical use of the LVC cement.

Thus, the Norwegian and Swedish hip registers and one RSA study have demonstrated inferior clinical results when hip prostheses are fixed

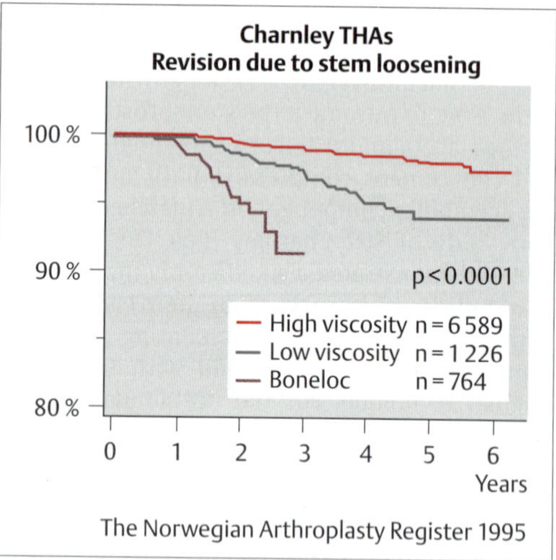

Fig. 2 Upgraded data on the survival of Charnley hips fixated with high viscosity, low viscosity and Boneloc cement. Presented with permission of the Norwegian Arthroplasty Register (Leif Havelin, MD).

with MMA-type bone cements of low viscosity. These results might be explained by sealing and pressurization difficulties during cementation and its use in the acetabulum with the patient

Table **1** The composition of Palacos R and Boneloc cement (from Thanner et al., Acta Orthopaedica Scandinavica 1995; 66: 207 – 14. With permission of the author and the Scandinavian University Press)

	Palacos®		Boneloc®	
Liquid				
Monomer	methyl methacrylate	97.8%	methyl methacrylate	50%
			decyl methacrylate	30%
			isobornyl methacrylate	20%
Accelerator	N,N-dimethyl-p-toluidine	2.1%	N,N-dimethyl-p-toluidine	0.5%
			dihydroxypropyl-p-toluidine	0.9%
Stabilizing agent	hydrokinon	65 ppm	hydrokinin-monomethyl ether	100 ppm
Color	chlorophyll		–	
Powder				
Polymer	methyl methacrylate-methyl acrylate	84.5%	methyl butyl methacrylate	90%
Contrast medium	zirconium oxide	15%	zirconium oxide	10%
Initiator	benzoyl peroxide	0.5%	benzoyl peroxide	0.7%
Color	chlorophyll	0.05%	Fd.&Blue No.2 Al.Lake	0.1%
Liquid/powder ratio	31/69		32/68	

positioned supine is particularly unsuitable. One controlled clinical trial could not demonstrate any difference between the two cement types but even in that study handling difficulties of the low viscosity cement were noticed.

Boneloc is a bone cement based on butyl methacrylate and which was introduced in 1990. Its composition is given in Table **1** and compared to that of Palacos R. Lowering both the exotherm and monomer leakage by using this bone cement was assumed to imply major advantages. Many laboratory tests were published by the group of innovators indicating no major differences in mechanical strength compared to conventional cement brands. However, no clinical trial was undertaken before marketing. Beginning in 1995, reports on an alarming number of early failures appeared (Riegels-Nielsen et al., 1995; Suominen, 1995; Nilsen and Wiig, 1996). Thanner et al. (1995) evaluated the chemical and mechanical properties of the cement and performed a randomized clinical study of 30 hips including RSA. They confirmed the lower curing temperature of Boneloc but compared to Palacos the tensile strength and Young's modulus were reduced. The glass transition temperature – an important parameter previously not fully taken into account – was 74 °C compared to 119 °C for Palacos. RSA during the first postoperative year revealed increased proximal migration of the cup and increased subsidence of the stem when Boneloc

had been used. Part of the stem subsidence occurred inside the cement mantle. All these reports, and what was found in the Norwegian register (Havelin et al., 1995), made the Norwegian Orthopaedic Society recommend stopping the use of Boneloc which thereafter was withdrawn from the market. Remarkably, the innovators own first 190 consecutive primary hips implanted with Boneloc cement and with a follow-up of 24–44 months were reported to perform clinically not differently from hips fixed with MMA cements. However, 20 per cent of the Exeter stems subsided more than 3 mm (Jensen et al., 1995). Klyver et al. (1996) could not demonstrate any difference between hip prostheses fixed with Simplex and Boneloc cements in their randomized study with a mean follow-up of 2.5 years. Only one revision had been performed in each group and in the radiographic evaluation no significant difference was observed regarding fixation pattern. However, only 97 hips were originally included implying a considerable risk of a type 2 error. According to the Company's instruction, Klyver et al. (1996) often discarded unsatisfactory mixes of cement which might not have been the case in the other studies. The authors therefore blame the mixing system rather than the Boneloc cement itself. They also hypothesize that their double tapered stem is better suited to combine with Boneloc cement than the Charnley type stems used in the other studies. This could fit with the unexpected somewhat lower survival of Charnley prostheses reported by the Norwegian register (Espehaug et al., 1995).

The handling characteristics of a bone cement is not only a question of whether it is of a high or low viscosity type. Storage temperature, type of mixing system, and the experience of the surgeon and the assisting nurse are also of importance. For example, storage of a high viscosity cement at 4 °C implies that the mixing procedure in syringes or bowls is simplified and that the mixture becomes more homogenous. The viscosity will also be reduced and injection of the cement and insertion of the prosthesis must therefore be postponed for about two minutes compared to a cement stored at room temperature.

Furthermore, it is obvious that the ability of the cement to penetrate into cancellous bone depends not only on the viscosity but also on how well the bone has been cleaned from debris and blood clots and how well the pressurization has counteracted the blood pressure. The bleeding can also be reduced by the use of hypotensive anesthesia, by lavage with freezing saline solution and, less effectively, by adrenaline and hydrogen peroxide tamponades (Bannister et al., 1990). Precooling the metallic stem prosthesis does not influence bone temperature but prolongs the setting time of the cement (Toksvig-Larsen et al., 1991). Preheating the stem to 44 °C reduces the cement porosity close to the stem prosthesis while only neglibly increasing bone temperature. The setting time will be shortened (Bishop et al., 1996).

From this concise review it may be clear that a bone cement after mixing must result in a homogenous product of low porosity and which is easy to introduce both in the acetabulum and in the femoral canal. It is of utmost importance to get familiar with the behaviour of *one* brand and under various circumferential conditions. However, it seems from the literature as if bone cements of low viscosity have performed inferiorly. Handling difficulties and a longer "learning curve" are the most likely reasons but for Boneloc and LVC also unsatisfactory physical properties. It must also be strongly warned against new bone cements which have not been evaluated in clinical trials. Even if their chemical and physical properties may seem attractive, history has taught us that a too early introduction on the market may become an expensive lesson.

References

Bannister GC, Young SK, Baker AS, Mackinnon JG, Magnusson PA. Control of bleeding in cemented arthroplasty. J Bone Jt Surg 1990; 72 B (3): 444 – 6.

Barrack RL, Mulroy RD, Harris WH. Improved cementing techniques and femoral component loosening in young patients with hip arthroplasty. J Bone Jt Surg 1992; 74 B (3): 385 – 9.

Bishop NE, Ferguson S, Tepic S. Porosity reduction in bone cement at the cement-stem interface. J Bone Jt Surg 1996; 78 B (3): 349 – 56.

Carlsson ÅS, Nilsson J-Å, Blomgren G, Josefsson G, Lindberg LT, Önnerfält R. Low- vs. high-viscosity cement in hip arthroplasty. Acta Orthop Scand 1993; 64 (3): 257 – 62.

Davies JP, Jasty M, O'Connor DO, Burke DW, Harrigan TP, Harris WH. The effect of centrifuging bone cement. J Bone Jt Surg 1989; 71 B: 39 – 42.

Espehaug B, Havelin L, Engesaeter LB, Vollset SE, Langeland N. Early revision among 12,179 hip prostheses. Acta Orthop Scand 1995; 66 (6): 487 – 93.

Granhed H, Malchau H, Herberts P, Johansson O. A 7 – 9-year follow-up of THR operated on with low viscosity cement. Acta Orthop Scand 1991; 62: (Suppl. 246).

Havelin L, Espehaug B, Vollset SE, Engesaeter LB. The effect of the type of cement on early revision of Charnley total hip prostheses. A review of eight thousand five hundred and seventy-nine primary arthroplasties from the Norwegian Arthroplasty Register. J Bone Jt Surg 1995; 77 A (10): 1543 – 50.

Jensen JS, Bødtker S, Kramhøft M, Thomsen PB, Petersen D, Nielsen K. Clinical results after 2 – 4 years with a new MMA/DMA/IBMA bone cement used for fixation of the femoral stem. Hip International 1995; 5 (1): 31 – 6.

Klyver H, Jacobsen K, Kofoed H. Boneloc versus Simplex cement for fixation of femoral components. An interim report of a prospective randomized study of THRs with a 2.5-year mean follow-up time. Hip International 1996; 6 (3): 112 – 8.

Miller J, Burke DL, Krause W, Ahmed A, Kelebay L, Tremblay G. Improved fixation of knee arthroplasty components by the injection of acrylic cement into cancellous bone surfaces. J Bone Jt Surg 1979; 61 B (4): 515.

Mjöberg B, Franzén H, Selvik G. Early detection of prosthetic-hip loosening. Comparison of low- and high-viscosity bone cement. Acta Orthop Scand 1990; 61 (3): 273 – 4.

Mulroy RD, Harris WH. The effect of improved cementing techniques on component loosening in total hip replacement. An 11-year radiographic review. J Bone Jt Surg 1990; 72 B: 757 – 60.

Nilsen AR, Wiig M. Total hip arthroplasty with Bone-loc®: loosening in 102/157 cases after 0.5 – 3 years. Acta Orthop Scand 1996; 67 (1): 57 – 9.

Noble PC, Swartz E. Penetration of acrylic bone cements into cancellous bone. Acta Orthop Scand 1983; 54: 566 – 73.

Önsten I, Besjakov J, Carlsson ÅS. Improved radiographic survival of the Charnley prosthesis in rheumatoid arthritis and osteoarthritis. Results of new versus old operative techniques in 402 hips. J Arthroplasty 1994; 9 (1): 3 – 8.

Riegels-Nielsen P, Sørensen L, Andersen HM, Lindequist S. Boneloc® cemented total hip prostheses. Acta Orthop Scand 1995; 66 (3): 215 – 7.

Roberts DW, Poss R, Kelley K. Radiographic comparison of cementing techniques in total hip arthroplasty. J Arthroplasty 1986; 1: 241 – 7.

Russotti GM, Coventry MB, Stauffer RN. Cemented total hip arthroplasty with contemporary techniques. A five-year minimum follow-up study. Clin Orthop 1988; 235: 141 – 7.

Suominen S. Early failure with Boneloc® bone cement. 4/8 femoral stems loose within 3 years. Acta Orthop Scand 1995; 66 (1): 13.

Thanner J, Freij-Larsson C, Kärrholm J, Malchau H, Wesslén B. Evaluation of Boneloc®. Chemical and mechanical properties, and a randomized clinical study of 30 total hip arthroplasties. Acta Orthop Scand 1995; 66 (3): 207 – 14.

Toksvig-Larsen S, Franzén H, Ryd L. Cement interface temperature in hip arthroplasty. Acta Orthop Scand 1991; 62 (2): 102 – 5.

The Cemented Prostheses: What is Sure, What is Open?

J. Schmidt

Introduction

Since the introduction of cemented total hip arthroplasties by Charnley in 1960 the results for the loosening-free survival of the implants has dramatically improved. From 24% failures after 6 years the failure rate has decreased to less than 2% after 7 to 8 years in specialized institutions. More obvious is this in the Sweden Study (Malchau and Herberts, 1996) based on 92,017 cemented implantations considering all patients and institutions in one country with a decreased failure rate from 23.2% after 15 years for the implantations from 1978–1983 to 8.1% after 10 years for implantations from 1984–1989, and now 1.6% after 3 years for implantations from 1990 to 1994. Due to these excellent results the total hip arthroplasty is a standardized operation with 120 000 implantations in Germany each year. About 60–80% are cemented stems and about 40% cemented cups.

To answer the question of the title is very difficult and may be subjectively. Additionally, publications dealing with techniques and problems of cementation are predominantly concerning the stem. So the answer will be focused only on the stem implantation.

What is Sure?

Distal intramedullary plugging improves the cement quality and reduces the risk of failure (Oh et al., 1978; Harris and McGann, 1986; Poss et al., 1988; Weber, 1988; Malchau and Herberts, 1996). Centralizing of the stem and its correct axis reduces the shear strength in the cement with a reduction of cement-cracking and therefore a reduction of loosening (Svensson et al., 1977; Gruen et al., 1979; Willert, 1991; Kahl et al., 1993). Also voids in the cement mantle are a risk for cement-cracking and should be reduced (Lidgren et al., 1984; Poss et al., 1988; Draenert, 1989; Harris and McGann, 1986) and there was

no doubt in Europe that it can be achieved best by a vacuum mixing technique. Nevertheless, this could not be confirmed in the recent study of Malchau and Herberts (1996), probably due to the different vacuum mixing systems which are now in use. Sharp corners, grooves, and groins on the stem are the reason for high shear strength and should be avoided (Svensson et al., 1977; Kahl et al., 1993). The preparation of the femoral canal with brushes, lavage, or adrenaline-soaked sponges before the insertion of the cement improves the penetration of the cement into the cancellous bone (Harris et al., 1986; Poss et al., 1988).

In recent years the fat embolic syndrome became of interest for total hip arthroplasty (Hofmann et al., 1995) especially concerning cemented stems (Ulrich et al., 1986; Draenert, 1989; Schmidt et al., 1996). We know that we need a sufficient drainage to reduce the intramedullary pressure. This can be either achieved by the vacuum cementing technique (Draenert, 1989) or the 1991 introduced transprosthetic drainage system (Fig. 1) with a significant reduction of the intramedullary pressure (Schmidt, 1996).

What is Open?

There is discussion about the thickness of the cement mantle: Poss et al. (1988) prefer a complete filling of the femoral canal, called "white out" while Draenert (1989) tries to achieve a deep penetration of the cement into the cancellous bone. On the other hand, Jansson et al. (1993) showed that a thickness of more than 2–3 mm increases the shear strength whereas Sih and Connelly (1980) fear heat degeneration when the thickness exceeds 5 mm. Great discussion deals at the moment with the material. According to recent publications (Brien et al., 1992; Willert et al., 1996) titanium does not seem to be an ideal material for cemented stems and has an increased risk of early failures. On the other hand, this material

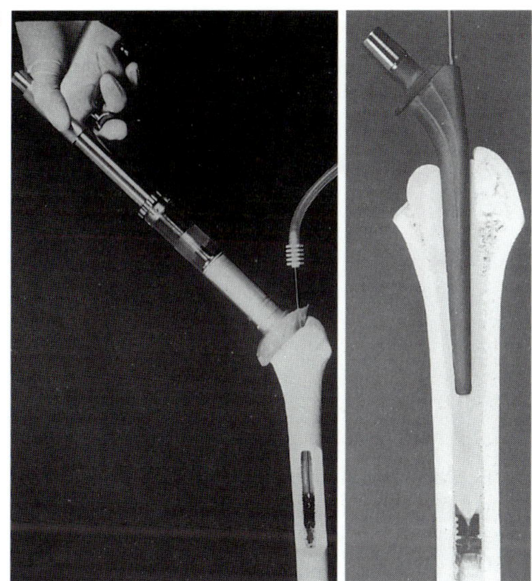

Fig. **1**   The transprosthetic drainage system (TDS): A drainage cannula is fixed in the center of a PMMA plug. A vacuum is applicated to the cannula. The cement will be suctioned into the femoral canal (**a**). Then a cannulated stem is pushed over the cannula working as a sufficient drainage until the final position of the stem is achieved and as a centralizing device (**b**). The cannula will be removed after curing of the cement.

has been in use since nearly 20 years in different designs and there are reports of excellent results (Nizard et al., 1992). Most of the cemented stems are matt, but there are superior results known with polished stems compared to a matt stem of the same design (Malchau and Herberts, 1996).

Also still open is the question of collar or collarless stems.

Own Results

On account of our previously published experimental results, we started a prospective study in 1994 with the transprosthetic drainage system and the TRIOS stem to evaluate the cement quality and the reduction of fat embolic syndrome. The diagnosis of the first 113 patients is shown in Figure **2.** We compared the anesthesiological parameters with the successive last 100 implantations of a cemented stem with a second-gen-

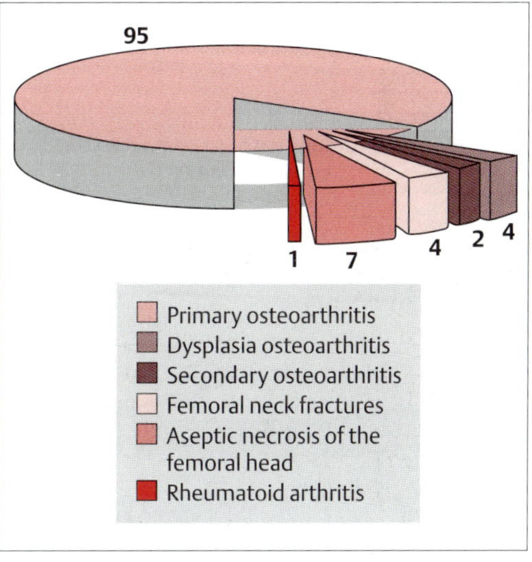

Fig. **2**   Diagnosis of the first 113 implantations with the TRIOS stem.

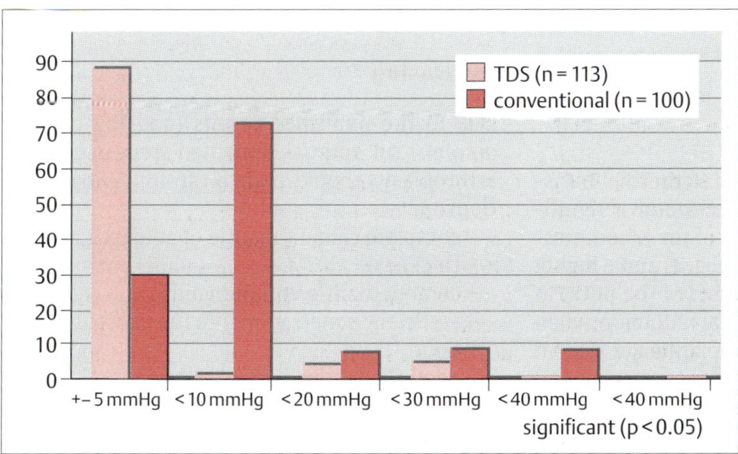

Fig. **3**   Anesthesiological evaluation of decreases of the blood pressure during application of the cement and the stem.

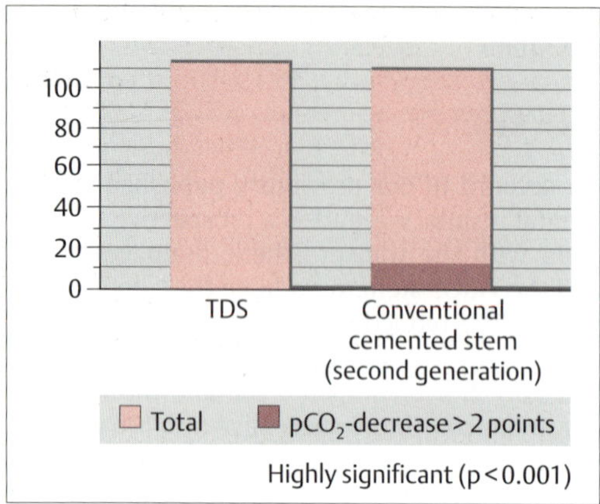

Fig. 4   Anesthesiological evaluation of the decrease of pCO_2 during application of the cement and the stem.

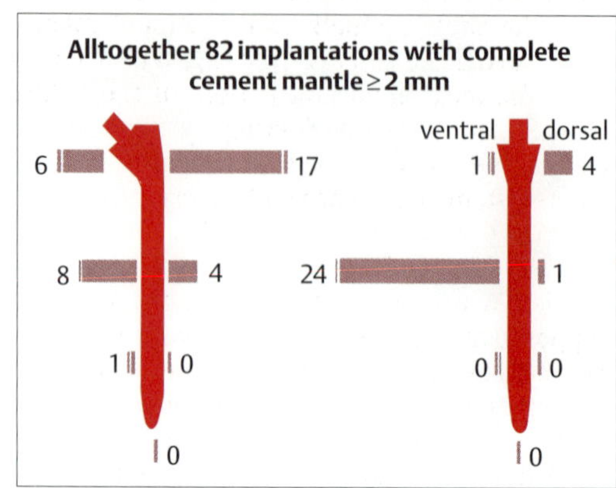

Fig. 6   Radiological evaluation of the thickness of the cement mantle.

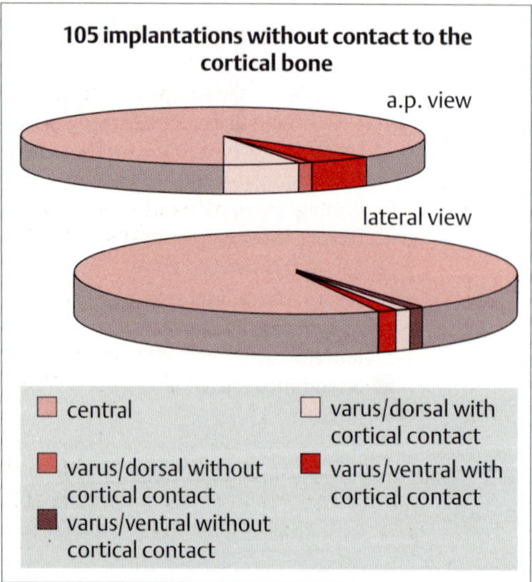

Fig. 5   Radiological evaluation of the stem position and the cement mantle.

eration cementing technique. With the transprosthetic drainage system we found a significant reduction of the decrease of the blood pressure during the implantation (Fig. 3) and a highly significant reduction of decreases of the pCO_2. In fact, there was no case of pCO_2 reduction when performing the transprosthetic drainage system (Fig. 4). As a result of the previous experimental trials and this clinical investigation, the transprosthetic drainage system is held to be highly effective to avoid fat embolic complications.

The postoperative result was documented with X-rays in a standardized anterior-posterior and lateral view. The evaluation showed 105 implantations with a completely intact cement mantle and a correct positioning (Fig. 5), but only 82 implantations with a complete cement mantle of at least 2 mm (Fig. 6). This result showed the centralizing effect of the drainage canula but can obviously be improved with an additional proximal centralizing device.

Considering these facts, the cement quality could be improved with the TRIOS stem, but we found an increased number of aseptic loosenings with this stem after 14–30 months. Due to this result we stopped the implantation of the TRIOS stem. A new stem will be developed considering all the experience we have obtained with our experiments, our prospective study, and the multicenter study.

Conclusion

Due to the published results (and my personal opinion), an optimal cemented stem in total hip arthroplasty should realize the following conditions:

- complete cement mantle of at least 2 mm thickness,
- cement mantle without voids,
- sufficient penetration into the cancellous bone,
- central position of the stem, and
- avoid embolic complications.

The first four conditions have the main aim to reduce the shear strength in the cement mantle and to avoid the cement-cracking, which seems to be the most important reason for the failure of cemented stems. Considering these conditions, we achieve excellent long-term results with cemented stems which are still superior to the results of cementless stems. The last point deals with the fat embolic syndrome, an intraoperative problem which was recently mostly neglected or supposed to be a problem of the anesthesiologist, but the fat embolic syndrome is a problem of the orthopedic surgeon. The surgeon can prevent the problem by a sufficient drainage of the femoral canal during the application of the cement and the insertion of the stem. The anesthesiologist has nearly no effective therapy if the fat embolic syndrome occurs.

References

Brien WW, Salvati EA, Betts F, Bullough P, Wright T, Rimnac C, Buly R, Garvin K. Metal levels in cemented total hip arthroplasty. Clin Orthop Rel Res 1992; 276: 66 – 74.

Draenert K. Modern cementing techniques. Acta Orthop Belgica 1989; 55 – 3: 273 – 93.

Gruen TA, McNeice GM, Amstutz H. "Modes of Failure" of cemented stem-type femoral components. Clin Orthop Rel Res 1979; 141: 17 – 26.

Harris WH, McGann WA. Loosening of the femoral component after use of the medullary plug cementing technique. J Bone Joint Surg (Am) 1986; 68: 1064 – 6.

Hofmann S, Huemer G, Kratochwill C, Kolle-Strametz J, Hopf R, Schlag G, Salzer M. Pathophysiologie der Fettembolie in der Orthopädie und Traumatologie. Orthopäde 1995; 24: 84 – 93.

Jansson V, Zimmer M, Kühne HJ, Ishida A. Blutschlieren im Knochenzement – Einfluß der Zementiertechnik. Unfallchirurg 1993; 96: 390 – 4.

Kahl S, Kranz C, Kuhlbach M. Einfluß von Zementierungsfehlern auf die mechanische Beanspruchung des Knochenzementes. Biomed Technik 1993; 38: 298 – 302.

Lidgren I, Drar H, Möller J. Strength of polymethylmethacrylate increased by vacuum mixing. Acta Orthop Scand 1984; 55: 536 – 41.

Malchau H, Herberts P. Prognosis of total hip replacement. 63 rd Annual Meeting of American Academy of Orthopaedic Surgeons, Atlanta, USA, 1996.

Nizard RS, Sedel L, Christel P, Meunier A, Soudry M, Witvoet J. Ten years survivorship of cemented ceramic-ceramic total hip prosthesis. Clin Orthop Rel Res 1992; 282: 53 – 63.

Oh I, Carlson CE, Tomford WW, Haris WH. Improved fixation of the femoral component after total hip replacement using a methacrylate intramedullary plug. J Bone Joint Surg (Am) 1978; 60: 608 – 13.

Poss R, Walker P, Spector M. Strategies for improving fixation of femoral components in total hip arthroplasty. Clin Orthop Rel Res 1988; 235: 181 – 93.

Schmidt J, Specht R, Steür G. Advantage of the transprosthetic drainage system (TDS) for application in cemented hip arthroplasty – a standardized experimental comparison with other cementing techniques. Arch Orthop Trauma Surg 1996; 115: 153 – 7.

Schmidt J. Das transprothetische Drainagesystem zur optimierten Zementierung von Hüftendoprothesenschäften. Operat Orthop Traumatol 1996; 8: 239 – 42.

Sih GC, Connelly GM. The effect of thickness and pressure on the curing of PMMA bone cement for the total hip joint replacement. J Biomechanics 1980; 13: 347 – 52.

Svensson NL, Valliappan S, Woods RD. Stress analysis of human femur with implanted Charnley prosthesis. J Biomechanics 1977; 10: 581 – 8.

Ulrich C. Stellenwert der Entlastungsbohrung zur Reduzierung der Knochenmarksausschüttung bei zementierten Hüftendoprothesen. Orthopäde 1995; 24: 138 – 43.

Weber BG. Pressurized cement fixation in total hip arthroplasty. Clin Orthop Rel Res 1988; 232: 87 – 95

Willert HG. Ein neues Hüftgelenk-Endoprothesensystem für die Implantation mit Knochenzement. In: Neugebauer (ed.). Was gibt es Neues in der Medizin. Medizinisches Jahrbuch Bd. 6, Dr. Peter Müller Verlag, Wien, 1991: 3 – 15.

Willert HG, Brobäck LG, Buchhorn GH, Jensen PH, Köster G, Lang I, Ochsner P, Schenk R. Crevice corrosion of cemented titanium alloy stems in total hip replacements. Clin Orthop Rel Res 1996; 333: 52 – 75.

PMMA as a Drug Carrier

B. Nies

Implant materials based on **P**oly-**M**ethyl-**M**eth-**A**crylate (PMMA) have a long history as clinically used drug carriers and especially as antibiotic carriers.

Bone cements with antibiotics (e.g., Refobacin®-Palacos®) and the implantable local antibiotic carrier Septopal® have been routinely used for many years for the prophylaxis and therapy of local infections.

The attractivity of PMMA as drug carrier is based on a range of important properties, unmatched by other polymeric substances:
- excellent biocompatibility – bioinertness,
- high purity of PMMA and its derivatives,
- long history of use as implant material,
- good compatibility with many relevant drugs,
- good release properties for many drugs, and
- established production technology (for bone cements and implants).

In the development of PMMA-based bone cements and implants which contain one or more drugs, the following main points have to be considered:
- How is the target indication defined?
- What is the medical need for this indication?
- Which properties are relevant for the drug?
- Which properties are relevant for the carrier?
- How can the relevant properties be realized in the combination?

Questions reaching beyond implant development are:
- What are the requirements for implant registration in different countries?
- Which factors influence the economy of the product?

In Figure **1** the relative importance of mechanical and pharmacological properties of PMMA-based implant materials is shown schematically depending on indications. This consideration demonstrates that any optimization of drug-release

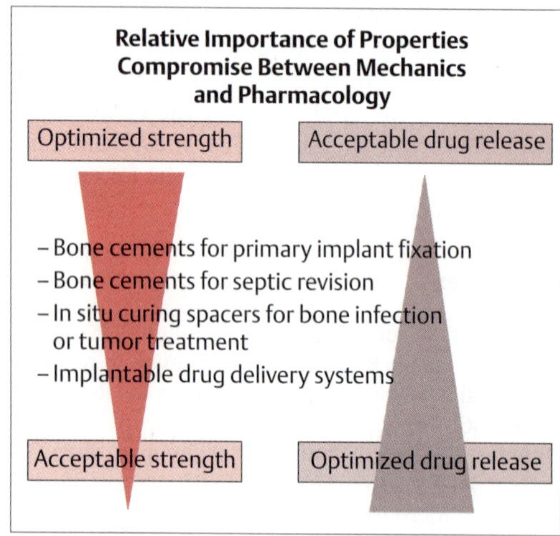

Fig. **1**   The use of PMMA as a drug carrier is dictated by the reciprocal relation of mechanical strength and pharmacological activity. Although this schematic drawing implies a direct correlation, a careful and intelligent selection within the range of properties of carrier material and drug and the technology to combine both, allows the design of an adequate product for the indicated target indications.

properties will influence the mechanical properties of the implant (e.g., bone cement) and it has to be the aim of the development process to find the most suitable compromise for a selected and defined indication.

An example is shown in Figure **2**. Refobacin®-Palacos® R is a bone cement mainly used for primary implant fixation. Among the gentamicin-containing bone cements Refobacin®-Palacos® R shows the highest antibiotic release. Nevertheless, the decrease in bending strength of approximately 6% compared to antibiotic-free Palacos® R is considered to be clinically non-relevant.

For a bone cement that contains gentamicin and clindamycin with highly improved antibacterial activity indicated for use in septic revision

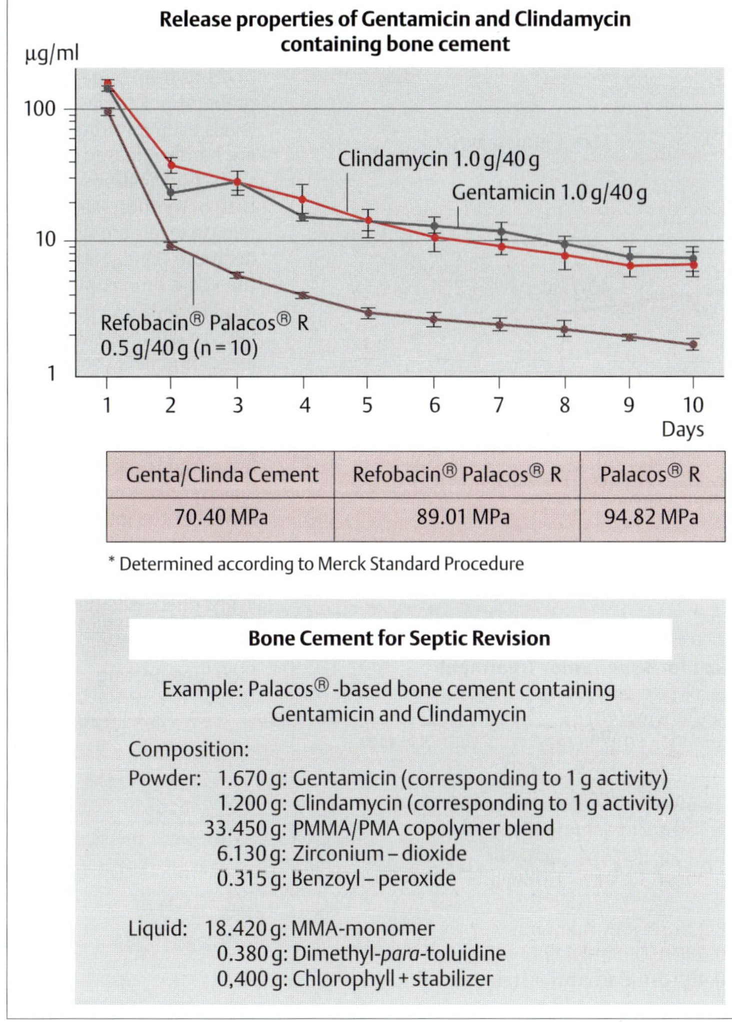

Genta/Clinda Cement	Refobacin® Palacos® R	Palacos® R
70.40 MPa	89.01 MPa	94.82 MPa

* Determined according to Merck Standard Procedure

Bone Cement for Septic Revision

Example: Palacos®-based bone cement containing
Gentamicin and Clindamycin

Composition:
Powder: 1.670 g: Gentamicin (corresponding to 1 g activity)
          1.200 g: Clindamycin (corresponding to 1 g activity)
         33.450 g: PMMA/PMA copolymer blend
          6.130 g: Zirconium – dioxide
          0.315 g: Benzoyl – peroxide

Liquid: 18.420 g: MMA-monomer
          0.380 g: Dimethyl-*para*-toluidine
          0,400 g: Chlorophyll + stabilizer

Fig. **2** The modification of Refobacin®-Palaocs® R that leads to the composition of this gentamicin and clindamycin containing bone cement results in a significantly increased drug release. As both these antibiotics act synergistically, the overall antimicrobial activity is greatly improved. The indicated values of bending strength measurements are considered to represent acceptable mechanical properties for a bone cement designed for application in septic revision.

arthroplasty, the release of both these drugs was adjusted to a much higher level. In this case the mechanical properties decline by ca. 20 % compared to Refobacin®-Palacos® R and 25 % relative to Palacos® R. For the antibacterial therapeutic use of Gentamicin/Clindamycin-Palacos® R, this compromise at the expense of bending strength is considered acceptable, especially as the value of 70.40 MPa is still well in excess of the 50 MPa required as the minimal value for antibiotic-free bone cements by the ISO standard (No. 5833).

An example going one step further in the direction of optimized pharmacological properties is the "Methotrexate Cement System", an *in situ* curing spacer designed for the treatment of primary and secondary bone tumors (Fig. **3**). The drug release in this system is adjusted by the application of two release modifiers – sodium carbonate added to the bone cement powder and methylpyrrolidone added to the cement liquid during the mixing process. With this composition the release of methotrexate is increased by 1 to 2 orders of magnitude during the first 10 days compared to a bone cement with the same amount of drug but without any release modifier. The decreased bending strength is of less importance and the value of 55 MPa seems to be well acceptable for the selected indication.

From the general aspects and the selected examples it can be concluded that the PMMA bone

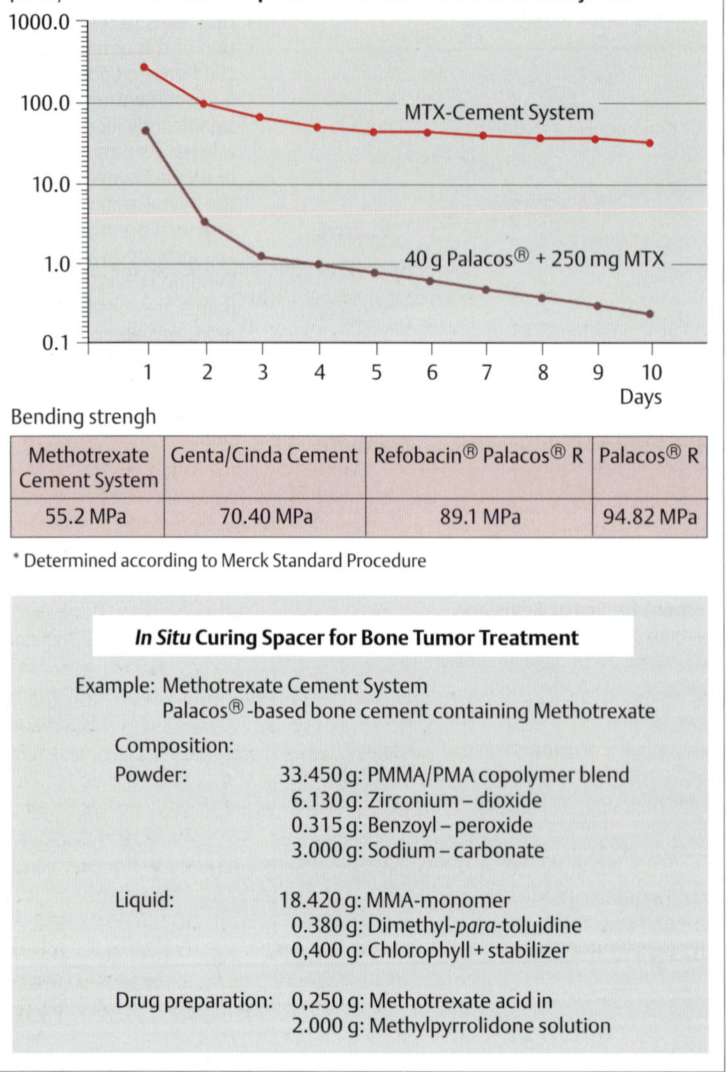

Bending strengh

Methotrexate Cement System	Genta/Cinda Cement	Refobacin® Palacos® R	Palacos® R
55.2 MPa	70.40 MPa	89.1 MPa	94.82 MPa

* Determined according to Merck Standard Procedure

In Situ Curing Spacer for Bone Tumor Treatment

Example: Methotrexate Cement System
Palacos® -based bone cement containing Methotrexate

Composition:
Powder: 33.450 g: PMMA/PMA copolymer blend
                       6.130 g: Zirconium – dioxide
                       0.315 g: Benzoyl – peroxide
                       3.000 g: Sodium – carbonate

Liquid: 18.420 g: MMA-monomer
                       0.380 g: Dimethyl-*para*-toluidine
                       0,400 g: Chlorophyll + stabilizer

Drug preparation: 0,250 g: Methotrexate acid in
                    2.000 g: Methylpyrrolidone solution

Fig. **3**   The use of suitable release modifiers allows to adjust the release profile of drugs from bone cement preparations to desired levels even for drugs that are hardly released without such modifications. In the case of methotrexate alone release levels are low and decrease rapidly, while at the same drug content a modified MTX-Cement System with the two release modifiers sodium carbonate and methylpyrrolidone shows a considerably higher drug release that is retained over an extended period of time. For the intended indication the determined bending strength is of less importance, albeit a value of 55.2 Mpa is still sufficient for applications with high load bearing.

cement system is very versatile in its applicability as a drug carrier. The adjustable range reaches from a bone cement with additional drug carrier function that can be designed to have high strength and still good drug release properties to *in situ* curing implantable drug delivery systems with excellent drug release properties and still acceptable mechanical behavior.

Among the different implant materials the PMMA-based drug carriers will retain their importance for those indications where the selection is based on mechanical properties and/or where a transitory implantation of a nonresorbable drug delivery system is indicated.

Pharmacological and Clinical Results with Gentamicin-PMMA Beads in Osteomyelitis

G. H. I. M. Walenkamp

Introduction

Gentamicin-PMMA beads are spherical balls of bone cement (methyl-methylmethacrylate copolymer) with a diameter of 7 mm and with 10, 30, or 60 beads strung together on a thread. The beads contain 7.5 mg of gentamicin sulfate, after implantation transformed to 4.5 mg of the active gentamicin base. In each bead 20 mg of zirconium dioxide, a little glycine, and a catalyzer are admixed.

These beads are the results of the experimental clinical work by Klaus Klemm, using handmade beads of gentamicin-admixed bone cement (Refobacine-Palacos®) in osteomyelitis (Klemm, 1993). Since they are now commercially available (Septopal®, E. Merck, Darmstadt) indications for use in all kinds of infections have been extended, and the use of suction drainage systems in orthopedic surgery has dramatically decreased.

After a period of 20 years using these gentamicin-PMMA beads, it is opportune to make a balance of their possibilities. To give an insight in the possibilities and limits of the beads pharmacokinetic data are helpful and provide an understanding of the clinical results.

Pharmacokinetics in Orthopedic Infections

To study the pharmacokinetics as well as the influence of a two weeks gentamicin load on the kidneys, about 1200 serum and urine samples in five patients were studied (Table **1**). The patients were operated twice: a debridement with implantation of 48–360 beads at $t = 0$, and an extraction of the beads at $t = 2$ weeks. In the serum the concentrations of gentamicin, creatinine, and β-2-microglobulin were measured. The renal excretion rates of creatinine (μmol/min), β-2-microglobulin (ng/min), and gentamicin (μg/min), the total amount of gentamicin excreted in the urine, as well as the *in vivo* half-life of gentamicin were calculated (Walenkamp, 1986).

We studied the renal excretion rate for gentamicin instead of the urine concentrations (as usually described in the literature), because the urine concentration varies greatly with the urine production. The β-2-microglobulin was measured because the renal excretion of this protein is a very sensitive parameter for the function of the proximal tubule cells. It is in the proximal tubulus where gentamicin is accumulated and causes damage to the tubulus cells. In cases of nephrotoxicity the first renal damage will be measurable in changes of the reabsorbtion at this site.

The *serum gentamicin concentrations* were only measurable in one patient with 360 implanted beads in the case of a revised infected total hip prosthesis (Fig. **1**): after a peak value in the first day of almost 2 μg/ml, a plateau level was reached under 1 μg/ml.

In the other patients the serum gentamicin concentrations remained unmeasurable, below the detection level of 0.15 μg/ml. They could, however, always be calculated, knowing the urine concentration and the renal clearance:

sex	age	diagnosis	N beads	implantation
F	28 yr	osteomyelitis tibia	48 beads	14 days
M	25 yr	osteomyelitis femur	90 beads	14 days
M	33 yr	osteomyelitis tibia	49 beads	10 days
M	21 yr	osteomyelitis femur	90 beads	14 days
M	67 yr	revision infected THP	360 beads	14 days

Table **1** Data of five patients treated with gentamicin beads and pharmaco-kinetically studied

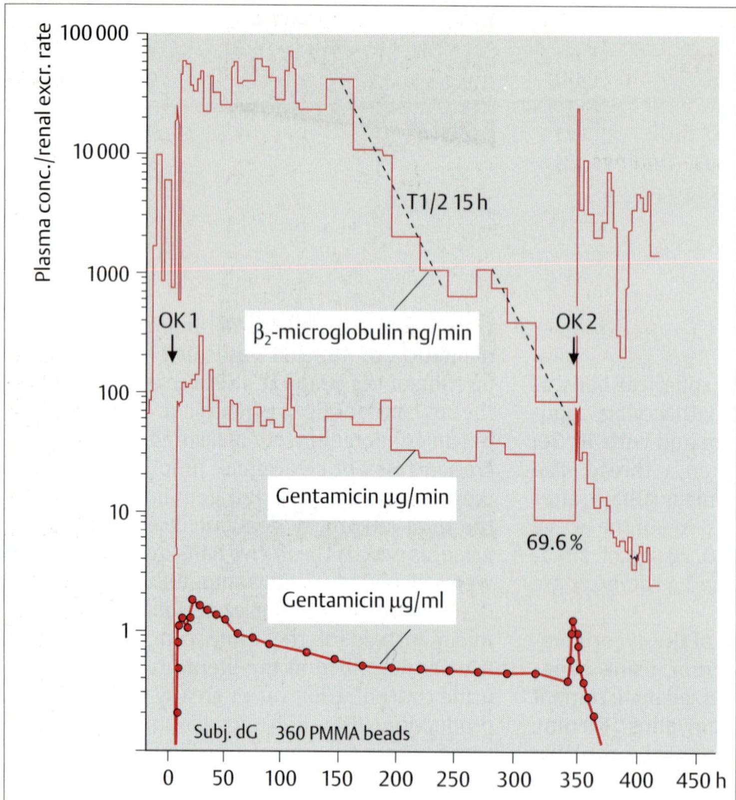

Fig. 1   A patient of 67 years with an infected THP was revised: after extraction and debridement 360 beads were implanted. In this patient, with a normal renal function, the serum gentamicin concentration was measurable during the whole implantation period. The graph shows a constant serum level during this two-week period, parallel to the renal excretion rate of gentamicin. The renal excretion rate of β-2-microglobulin fluctuates due the operation trauma, not to the gentamicin treatment.

Serum gentamicin concentration = renal excretion rate/renal clearance. The calculated serum gentamicin concentration was 0.03 – 0.4 μg/ml in the other patients treated with 48 – 90 gentamicin beads.

The *renal excretion rate of gentamicin* was remarkably constant during the whole treatment period of two weeks, at a level of 3 – 40 μg/min. The constant renal excretion reflects the constant elution of gentamicin out of the beads, resulting in the constant serum concentration as well. Hence, serum gentamicin concentrations and renal excretion curves are parallel (Fig. 1).

The *renal excretion of β-2-microglobulin* was only increased by the trauma of the operation, not by the constant gentamicin load on the renal tubule during the two weeks. The same holds true for the glomerular function: the clearances of creatinine and gentamicin did not increase. Thus, from these measurements we can conclude that no nephrotoxicity is measurable, and that the diffusion from the beads results in a constant

excretion of the gentamicin out of the body. In the period of measurement, these patients excreted in their urine 20 – 70% of the gentamicin implanted, resulting in an *in vivo half-life* of 6 – 10 days. This $t_{1/2}$ seems to be influenced by the vascularity of the surrounding tissues: excretion is faster when the beads are placed in muscles than in sclerotic bone.

Pharmacokinetics in Renal Impairment

It is not infrequent that patients have impaired renal function when they must be treated for orthopedic infections caused by sepsis or high age. The question is if gentamicin administration by beads may further affect the renal function. We therefore frequently check the gentamicin concentrations when patients appear to have a renal impairment.

We described a first patient in 1981 (Walenkamp, 1981). She had a creatinine clearance of 1 ml/min, necessitating hemodialysis. There were 150 gentamicin beads implanted, and a plateau level for serum gentamicin of about 3 µg/ml, slightly reduced to about 2 µg/ml by the hemodialysis, was measured. There was no accumulation of the gentamicin in spite of the impaired renal elimination. Since then these findings were confirmed in several other patients with renal functions of 10–50% of the normal. We have never found an increase of the gentamicin concentration, except in one patient.

This was a 64-year-old patient treated for an infected total knee prosthesis. After debridement and removal of the prosthesis, 300 beads were implanted (Fig. **2**). His creatinine clearance was at that moment about 15 ml/min, also influenced by the large operation with considerable blood loss. The serum gentamicin concentration increased in the first 5 postoperative days. Therefore, the nephrologist and clinical pharmacologist insisted on removal of the beads, but after removal it appeared that they had based their advice on the assumption that 600 beads were implanted (Fig. **3**), so we will never know if the removal was justified.

When another debridement was necessary one year later for an infected pseudarthrosis, 180 beads were implanted. The clearance at that moment was 30 ml/min. The renal function did not decrease, and a plateau level was seen between 1 and 2 µg/ml (Fig. **4**). The infection could be healed and consolidation of the comminuted femur and tibia into an arthrodesis was achieved.

Based on the measurements in about 10 renal-impaired patients we do not consider implantation of beads to be contraindicated in cases

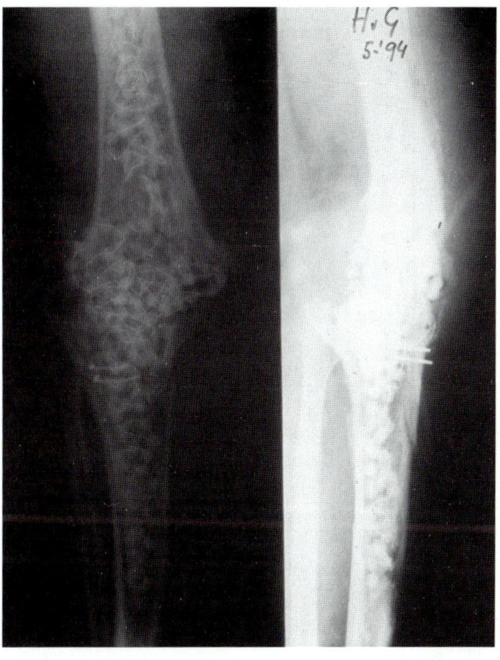

Fig. **2** In a 64-years-old patient a non-cemented knee prosthesis, infected but well fixed, was removed and 300 gentamicin beads implanted. He had a renal function of only 15%.

of renal impairment. Daily checks of the serum gentamicin concentration in the first week may show if a plateau level is reached, and at which level.

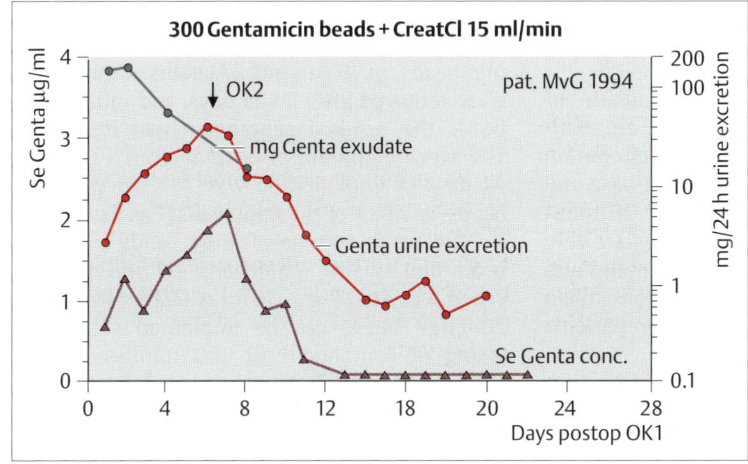

Fig. **3** After implantation of the 300 beads the serum gentamicin concentration increased and the beads were removed after 7 days. The gentamicin excreted in the urine of course parallels the serum gentamicin. The gentamicin released in the exudate is expressed as excreted mg gentamicin per day.

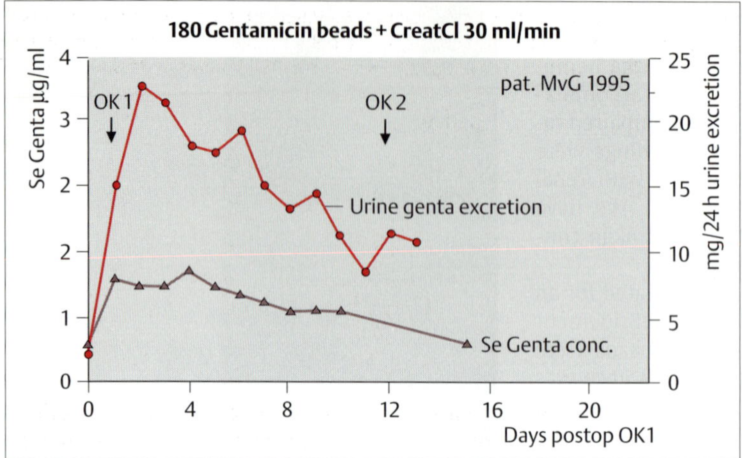

Fig. 4   One year later the same patient was treated again, and showed a plateau level for the serum gentamicin.

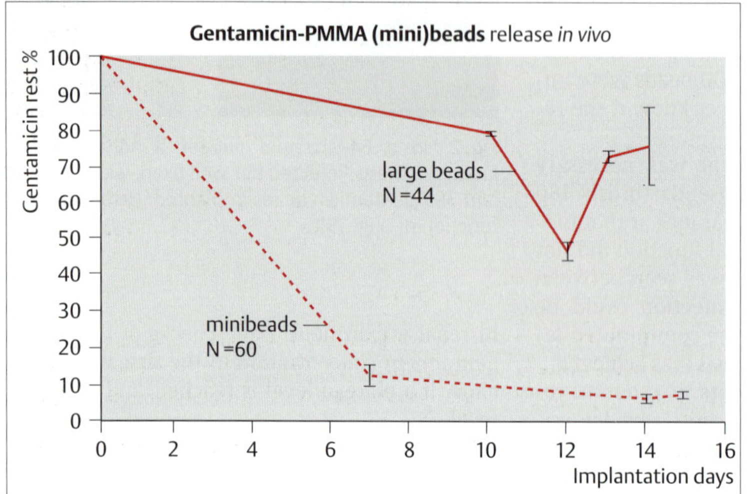

Fig. 5   The release in vivo of gentamicin out of large Septopal beads and minibeads, expressed as the percentage of the implanted amount of gentamicin. Gentamicin is released much better from minibeads.

Pharmacokinetics of Minibeads

When there is not sufficient room available for the beads of 7 mm diameter, minibeads are available. Their size is 3 × 5 mm, and they each contain the equivalent of 1.7 mg of gentamicin base and they are strung on chains with 10 or 20 minibeads. Developed for hand surgery, they are very useful as well in small osteomyelitic cavities and soft-tissue infections as well. Their gentamicin release in vivo was checked after use in patients (Walenkamp, 1989).

In 17 patients 19 chains were removed after 10 – 14 days of implantation. Of these, 44 beads were dissolved and the gentamicin left in the beads was measured.

The same procedure was performed with minibeads: in 19 patients 27 chains of minibeads were removed after 7 – 15 days, and in 60 minibeads the residual gentamicin was measured. The average amount of gentamicin release after 14 days of implantation was 24% for the large beads, and 93% of the minibeads (Fig. 5).

The mean volume of large beads is 0.5 ml/bead and of the minibeads 0.1 ml/minibead. When a cavity of, e.g., 10 ml is filled with beads, 20 large beads can be implanted containing 90 mg of gentamicin, or 100 minibeads with 179 mg of gentamicin. However, the release in two weeks of beads implanted in this 10 ml cavity will increase from 22 mg to 158 mg when minibeads are used instead of large beads. In

Table **2** History of results of different kinds of treatment for osteomyelitis. Modified after Schulitz (1982): results of 1950–1975 are based on a study of patients treated at the University of Heidelberg, the results of treatment with gentamicin beads in the literature (Vecsei, 1981; Klemm, 1988; Majid, 1985; Cierny, 1990) and our data

kind of treatment	period	healing quota
debridement	1950–1960	36%
debridement and saucerization and muscle transplantation	1958–1964	61%
saucerization and bone graft	1972–1975	85%
debridement and gentamicin beads	1977–1997	90–96%

general, the release is about seven times higher using minibeads. The explanation for this is that the release of the gentamicin from bone cement is a diffusion process that is related to the surface of the cement. A larger surface area results in an increased release. For the same reason the gentamicin release is much higher from beads when compared with a solid bone cement block, used as a spacer in prosthesis revision.

When a high concentration of gentamicin is needed, as in more resistent germs or very sclerotic bone, than minibeads shold be preferred instead of large beads, especially in small cavities.

Clinical Results

The treatment of osteomyelitis in the first 100 patients in our orthopedic department in Maastricht was evaluated with a follow-up of at least 1 year (mean 65 months).

In 78% of the patients the infection healed after one period of treatment. Such a treatment took 3 months maximally, and often contained several operations. The intervals between operations were always two weeks: if necessary several redebridements were performed and a reconstruction. The patients were operated, respectively, one time ($n = 60$), twice ($n = 15$), three times ($n = 2$), or five times ($n = 1$). In another 14% of the patients one or two other treatment periods for a relapse or a persistent infection were necessary to achieve healing. So the healing percentage increased up to 92%.

Survival analysis showed more relapses when the infection was very chronic (> 6 years), which was especially the case when they were referred by another orthopedic surgeon.

The relapses were seen mainly in the first and second year postoperatively. With increasing time postoperatively the chance for a relapse de-

creases such that we do not control the patients on a regular base when they are relapse-free for two years.

Comparison of these results with the literature is difficult because no survival analyses have been published before, and the series of osteomyelitis as published are very heterogenous. Results in other series of patients treated with beads report comparable healing percentages of 90–96% (Vecsei, 1981; Klemm, 1988; Majid, 1985; Cierny, 1990). There seems to be a gradual improvement in the results of osteomyelitis treatment in the last 40 years (Schulitz, 1982).

References

Cierny G. Chronic osteomyelitis: Results of treatment. In: Instructional Course lectures, Vol. 34. American Academy of Orthopaedic Surgeons. 1990: 495–508.

Klemm KW. Antibiotic bead chain. Clin Orthop 1993; 295: 63–76.

Majid SA, Lindberg LT, Gunterberg B, Siddiki MS. Gentamicin-PMMA beads in the treatment of chronic osteomyelitis. Acta Orthop Scand 1985; 56: 265–8.

Schulitz KP, Winkelmann W. Die Retrospektive eines großen Patientengutes mit chronischer Osteomyelitis der Jahre 1930–1975. In: Parsch K, Plaue R. (eds.). Hämatogene Osteomyelitis und posttraumatische Osteitis. Buchreihe für Orthopädie und orthopädische Grenzgebiete, Bd. 6 (ed. Schliegel KF). Medizinisch Literarische Verlagsgesellschaft mbH, Uelzen: 231–7.

Vecsei V, Barquet A. Treatment of chronic osteomyelitis by necretomy and gentamicin-PMMA beads. Clin Orthop Rel Res 1981; 159: 201–7.

Walenkamp GHIM, Vree TB. Treatment of a patient with impaired renal function with gentamicin-PMMA beads. Arch Orthop Traumat Surg 1981; 99: 137–41.

Walenkamp GHIM, Vree TB, van Rens ThJG. Gentamicin-PMMA beads. Pharmacokinetic and nephrotoxicological study. Clin Orthop 1986; 205: 171–83.

Walenkamp GHIM. Small PMMA beads improve gentamicin release. Acta Orthop Scand 1989; 60 (6): 668–9.

Clinical Results with PMMA Beads as an Antibiotic Delivery System

H. G. K. Schmidt, C. H. Siebert, S. Lösel

Introduction

The patients treated in the trauma department of the Berufsgenossenschaftlichen Unfallkrankenhaus Hamburg can be classified in three groups:
1. Accident victims treated primarily at our hospital. The osteomyelitis rate in our acutely injured patients was found to be 0.4%.
2. Patients transferred to us from other hospitals, frequently due to injuries requiring more extensive forms of treatment.
3. Patients with joint and/or bone infections after unsuccessful management in other units.

It must be pointed out, that the majority the cases of osteomyelitis and empyema seen in our hospital are difficult, if not extremely problematic. Simple infections are rarely treated.

In all cases with manifest soft-tissue, bone, and/or joint infections, gentamicin beads are used as a supportive measure as part of our standardized surgical revision protocol. Septopal® beads are also placed as a prophylactic measure in cases with open fractures and large soft-tissue injuries.

Our therapeutic regimen is naturally determined by the problem at hand, although we follow standardized guidelines. The treatment of bone infections consists of the following:

Primarily a radical removal of all dead bone and soft tissue, removal of unstable hardware and fracture stabilization is carried out. Should stability be given, cast splints are frequently applied to prevent the development of joint contractures. Skin defects are covered with artificial skin, such as Epigard®, as part of the first surgical debridement until a resolution of the infection can be obtained. Areas with bony defects are packed with antibiotic-loaded beads. These beads can also be placed subcutaneously to prevent a recurrence of the infection. Additionally, a systemic antibiotic treatment is carried out for 3 – 4 days.

After the resolution of the acute infection, which occurs, on average, in four weeks, the definitive management of the soft-tissue defect is carried out taking advantage of all the possibilities offered in the field of plastic surgery with a liberal use of various flaps. Bone defects are reconstructed step by step. Defects of up to 3 cm in shaft length are filled via autologous bone transplants. Larger defects require a distraction technique or a primary resection and shortening followed by secondary limb lengthening. Should autologous bone graft be used for the reconstruction, the defect should be filled stepwise or rather in layers, depending on the quality of the surrounding tissue. Immediately after the surgical revision, an early physical therapy program including all the various treatment forms should be enstated with partial weight bearing of 10 kg. The external fixators can be placed under tension in the course of treatment. Once bone stability has been achieved, load sharing orthopedic devices can be fitted – while still permitting only partial weight bearing of 10 kg (Figs. **1 a – j**).

Acute joint infections can be managed with repeated arthroscopic procedures combined with a systemic antibiotic treatment, possibly with a temporary placement of Septopal® beads into the joint. In cases with a chronic joint infection, per definition those existing for more than 7 days, a two-step open protocol is preferred. The first procedure is an urgent operation consisting of a double arthrotomy at the elbow, wrist, knee, or ankle joint, as well as a synovectomy, followed by a thorough lavage, drainage, and the implantation of gentamicin beads. The surgical wounds remain open after this procedure. The systemic antibiotic is chosen in accordance with the test result and administered for about five days (Figs. **2 a – g**).

In the days following this first operation, the patient and his open joint are placed in a bath

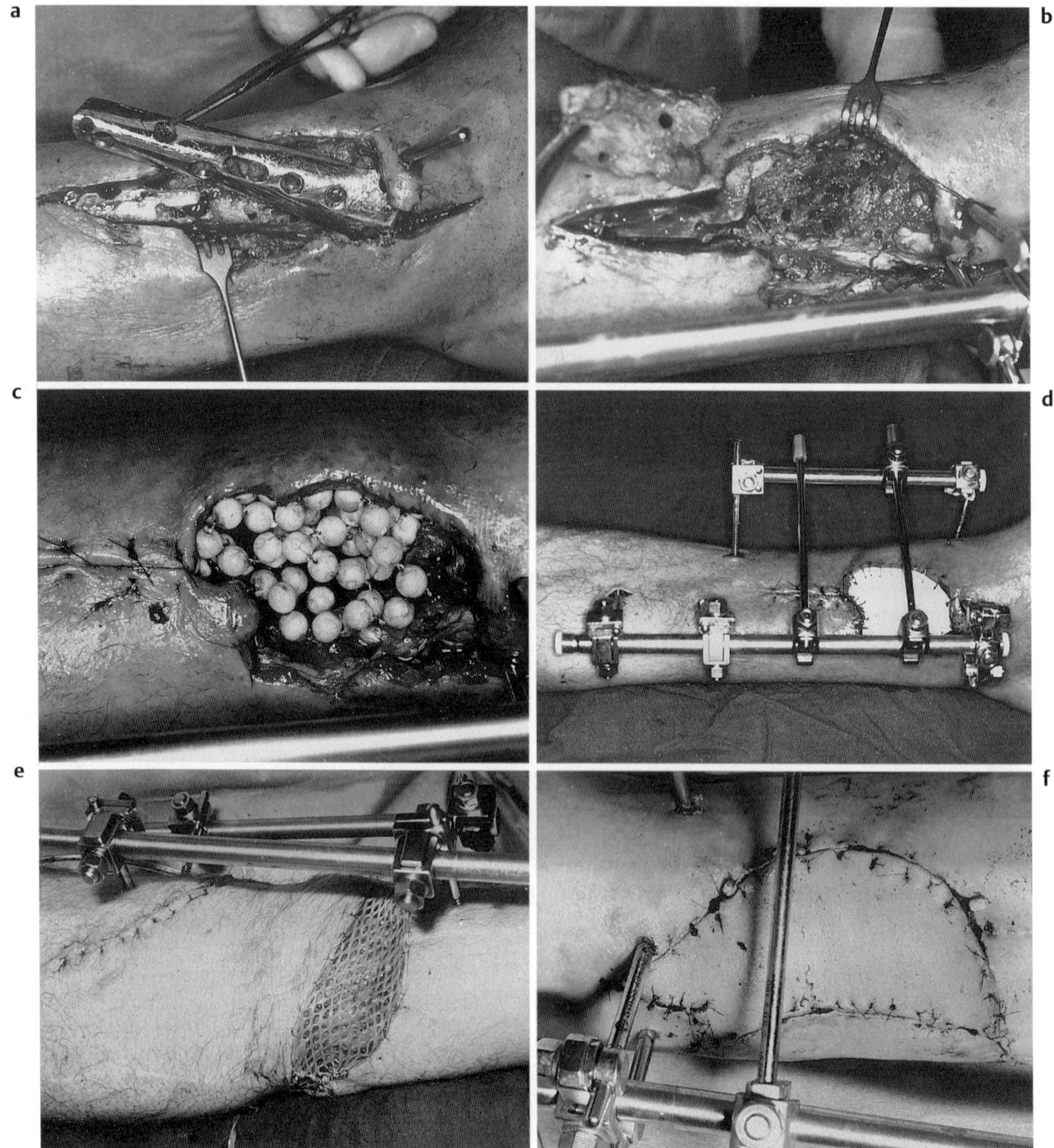

Fig. **1 a – d** Removal of the infected AO-plate in this case of a unstable distal tibial fracture, followed by a radical debridement, external fixation, insertion of Septopal® beads and wound closure with the help of Epigard®. **e + f** After 2 – 4 weeks, coverage of the soft tissue defect with a fasciocutaneous or free radial flap following renewed debridement in a second procedure can be carried out.

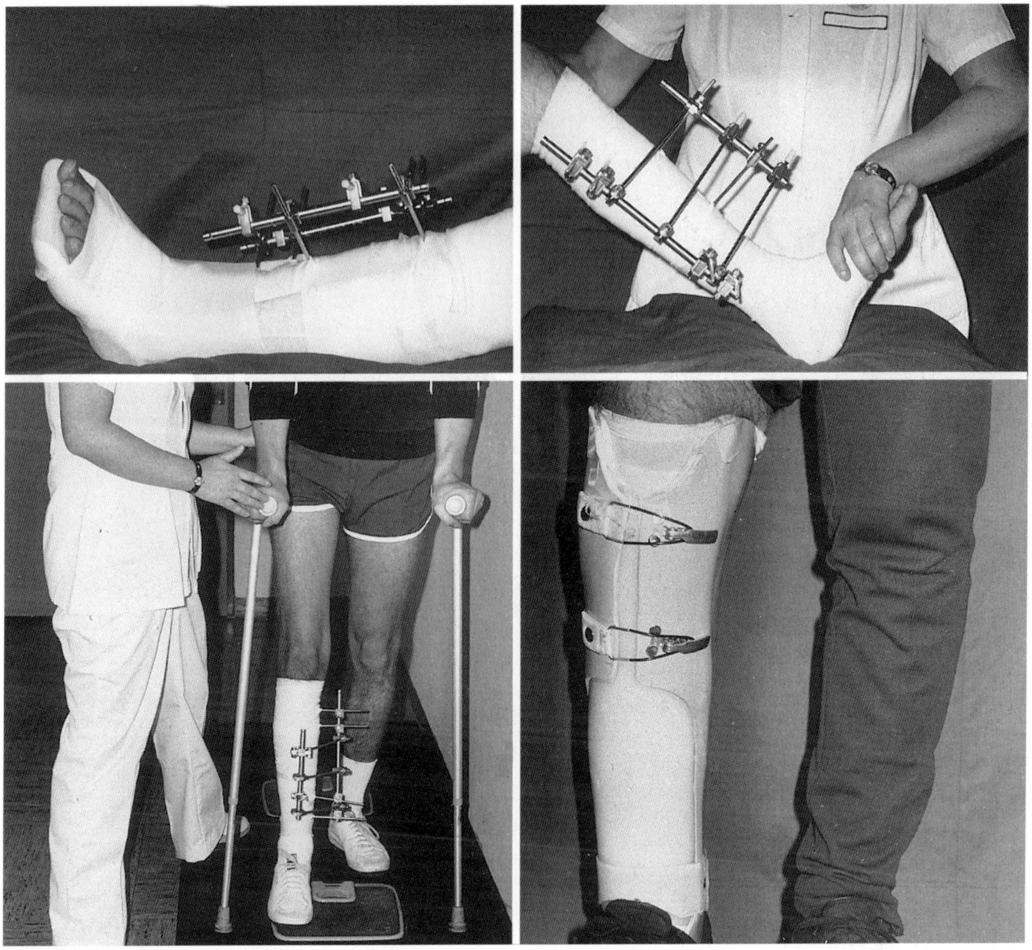

Fig. **1 g – j**   To avoid joint contractures a splint is used. Early onset of physical therapy with partial weight bearing (10 kg). Following fracture healing, a load sharing orthosis is fitted to avoid renewed fractures.

tub on a daily basis to irrigate the wound. The amount of wound secretion has to be monitored; should large amounts be registered, a renewed debridement of the joint is necessary. Has a cessation of the acute infection been achieved, the second operation can be carried out after seven to ten days, consisting of the removal of the beads, another debridement, joint lavage, and mobilization of the joint. Following a thorough lavage, the joint is closed over hemovac drains and mini-Septopal® beads, which are placed subcutaneously. An intensive physical therapy program including the use of passive motion machines or splints is then carried out (Figs. **2 h – l**).

In patients suffering from a combination of bone and joint infections, the described protocol can be adapted to suit the individual needs. In the following our treatment regimen will be demonstrated with the help of some exemplary cases.

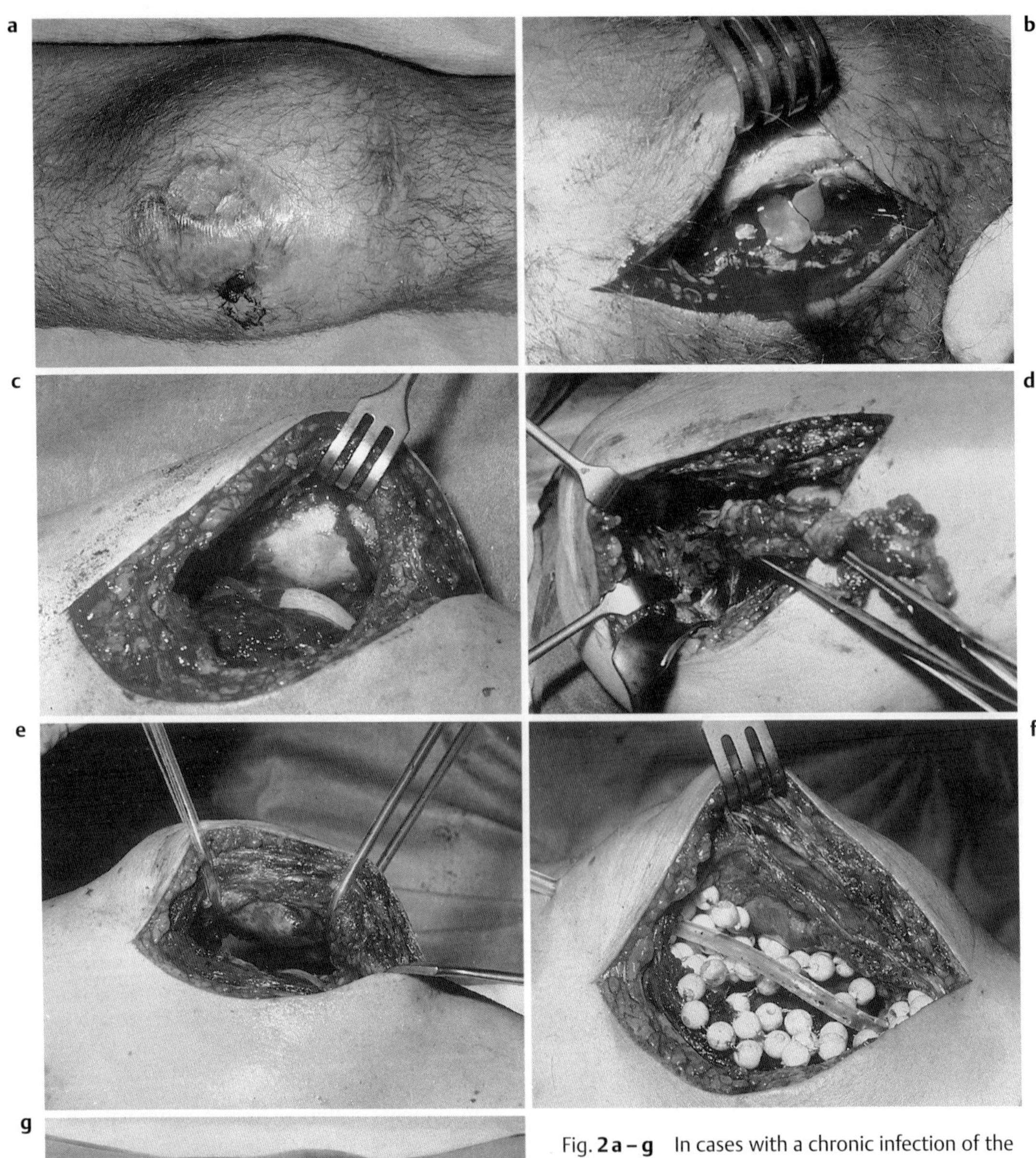

Fig. **2a – g** In cases with a chronic infection of the knee, the revision of the joint is carried out through a medial as well as lateral approach. Following the synovectomy, the joint is extensively irrigated, Septopal® beads are inserted, and the wounds are left open.

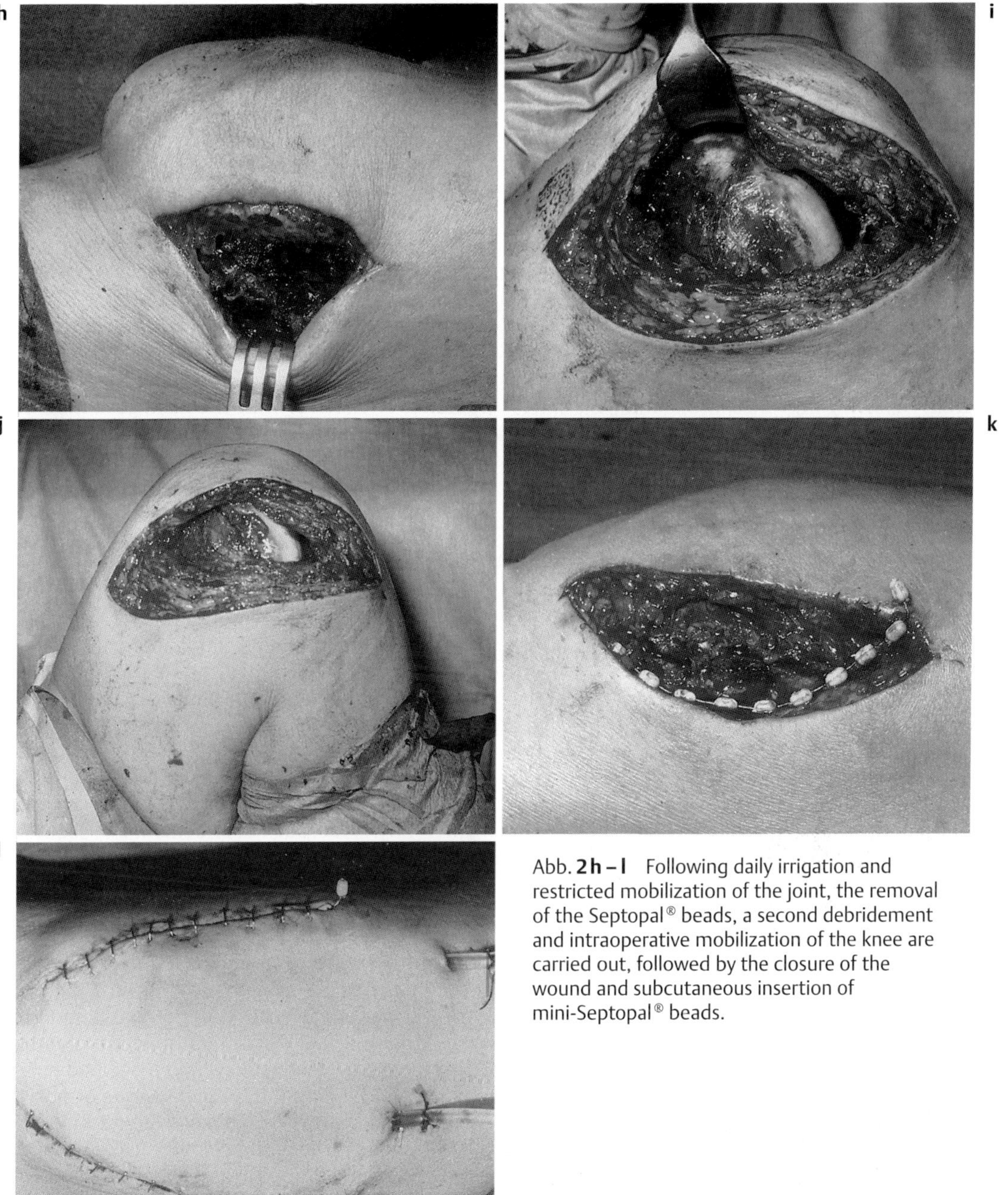

Abb. **2 h – l** Following daily irrigation and restricted mobilization of the joint, the removal of the Septopal® beads, a second debridement and intraoperative mobilization of the knee are carried out, followed by the closure of the wound and subcutaneous insertion of mini-Septopal® beads.

Case Reports

As an illustration for our form of infection prophylaxis, the case of a 25-years-old man with a third degree open tibial fracture with injury to the neurovascular bundle will be discussed. Following a radical debridement, the fracture was stabilized in an external fixator and the posterior tibial vessels were reconstructed. Gentamicin beads were placed in the bone defect and the skin defect was closed with Epigard®. In an infection-free state, seven days later, the conditioning of wound was begun. Two weeks later, the bone defect was filled with autologous bone and the soft-tissue defect closed with the help of a skin graft. Following fracture consolidation, the external fixator was removed after five months and a weight sharing orthosis was fitted. Full weight bearing was permitted after a total of nine months.

The second case is that of an acute osteomyelitis of the distal tibia following internal fixation with an AO plate without an associated empyema. The hardware removal, debridement, stabilization of the fracture zone in an external fixator without length correction, and the implantation of Septopal® beads was carried out as part of the first procedure. Once the infection calmed, length was restored to the tibia and the open reduction and internal fixation of the fibula, as well as an autologous bone transplantation, were performed. Physical therapy, tensioning of the fixator, full weight bearing after 5 months, fixator removal after 6 months and hardware removal from the fibula after 12 months were the next treatment steps. This patient was a colleague, who returned to private practice after 3 months with the fixator in place.

The third patient is a 45-year-old diabetic with a chronic osteomyelitis following plating of a distal tibial fracture associated with a soft-tissue defect. An infectious arthritis was not present. The hardware removal and extensive debridement led to an eight to ten cm long bone defect, which was temporarily packed with antibiotic beads. The soft-tissue defect was closed with the help of Epigard®. The intraoperative situation during the first procedure in 1985, a time during which the tissue was still stained with disulfine blue is depicted. Four weeks later, the acute infection resolved and the first bone graft was carried out. During the same procedure, soft-tissue closure was achieved with a free radial flap. Two further bone grafts were necessary to achieve a

full bone reconstruction. The fixator was loaded after 7 months and removed after 9 months. The result was an acceptable amount of function in the light of stable conditions. The X-ray three years after the completion of the treatment shows the outcome (Figs. **3 a – l**).

The following case reveals certain similarities, but the treatment took place in 1992, a point in time at which our protocol for large defects was changed to include distraction techniques. Once again a free radial flap was required for the closure of the soft-tissue defect. The bone defect amounted to eleven cm, the distraction time was 101 days and the consolidation time was 11 months. An unrestricted full weight bearing was possible after 18 months. The main advantage of the Ilisarow limb lengthening procedure is that an actual cortical cylinder results rather than a callus mass requiring secondary remodeling.

The next two case reports are exemplary for our treatment protocol as carried out in 1986, at which time bone defects of up to ten centimeteres were filled with autologous bone grafts. After 3 months, the external fixator was removed to shorten the immobilization period and replaced by an AO-plate. To reconstruct the bone defect, a total of four bone grafts as part of three different operations were necessary. In both cases, the patients were adolescents and the yield of the bone harvest was just enough to fill the defect. Since 1992 such cases are managed differently. A thorough debridement and sequesterectomy including the resection of the whole knee, which was also infected, led to a defect measuring 20 cm. In these instances, stability was achieved with the help of a ring fixator of the upper leg using an Italian system. After two weeks, a proximal osteotomy and callus distraction via two pulley wires is performed. To bridge the 20 cm defect a distraction time of 8 months was required. The fixator was removed after 18 months and replaced by a load-sharing orthosis. Full weight bearing was allowed after 8 months. The unstable docking site did not cause problems and represented a neoarthros with painless micromotion (Figs. **4 a – l**).

With the final examples, the treatment regimen for patients with a combined bone and joint infection is to be outlined. The first instance represents an infection of the hindfoot leading to bone necrosis in the calcaneus, parts of the talus, the navicular, cuboid, and cunieform bones. Following the sequestrectomy and tissue staining, stabilization was achieved with a modified ven-

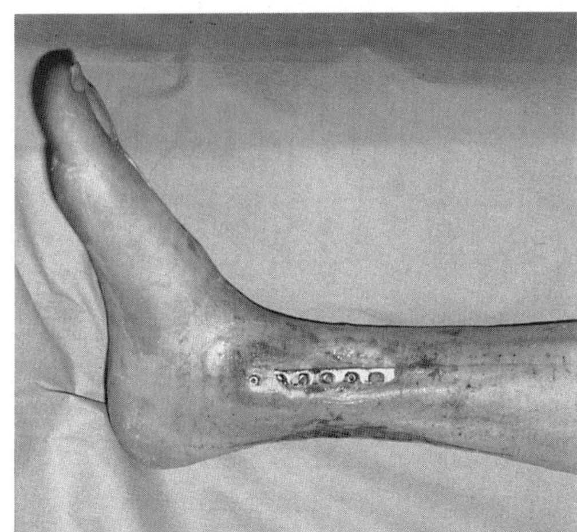

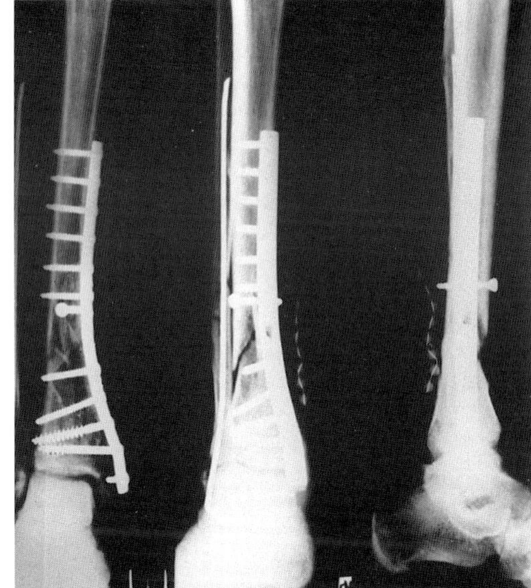

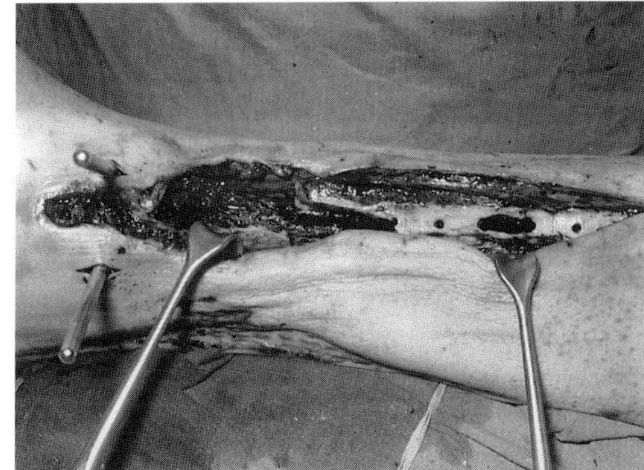

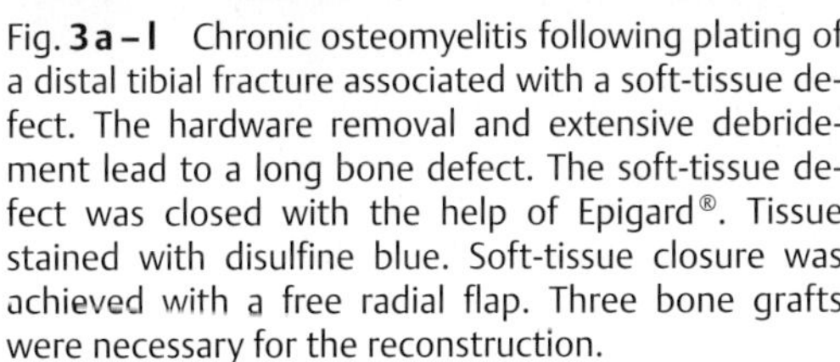

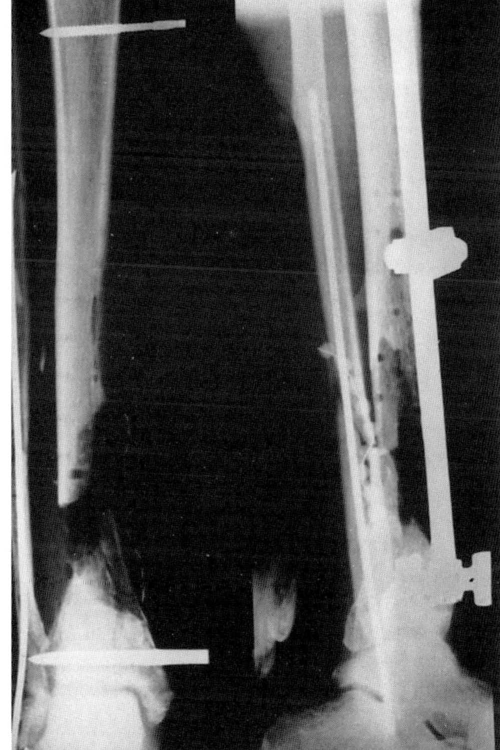

Fig. **3a–l** Chronic osteomyelitis following plating of a distal tibial fracture associated with a soft-tissue defect. The hardware removal and extensive debridement lead to a long bone defect. The soft-tissue defect was closed with the help of Epigard®. Tissue stained with disulfine blue. Soft-tissue closure was achieved with a free radial flap. Three bone grafts were necessary for the reconstruction.

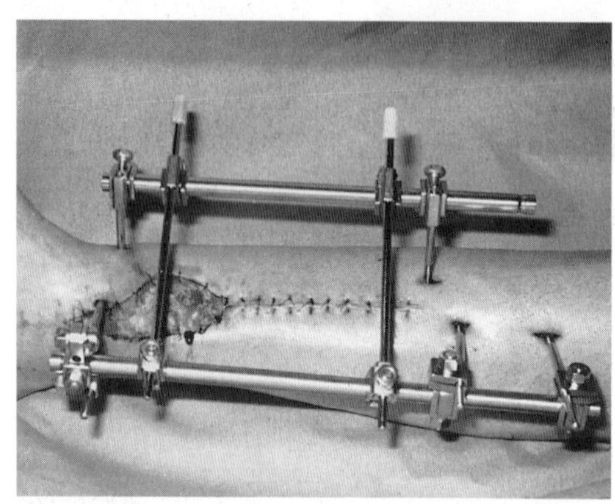

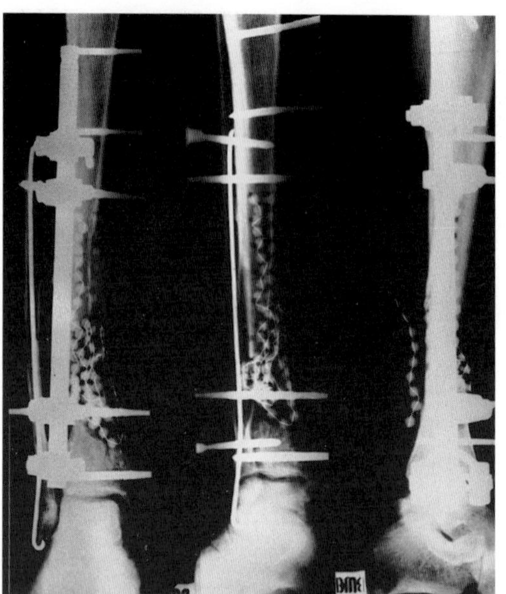

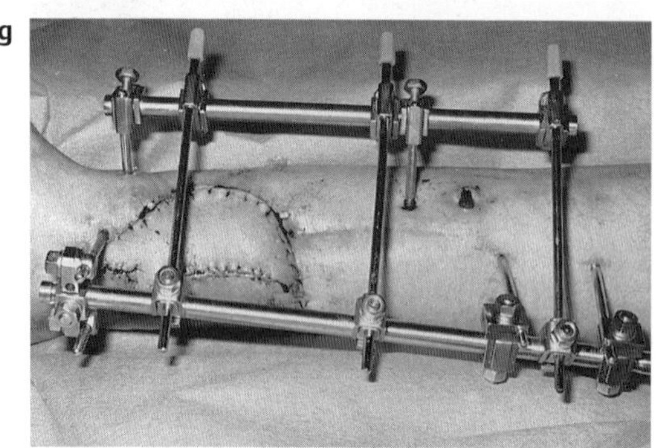

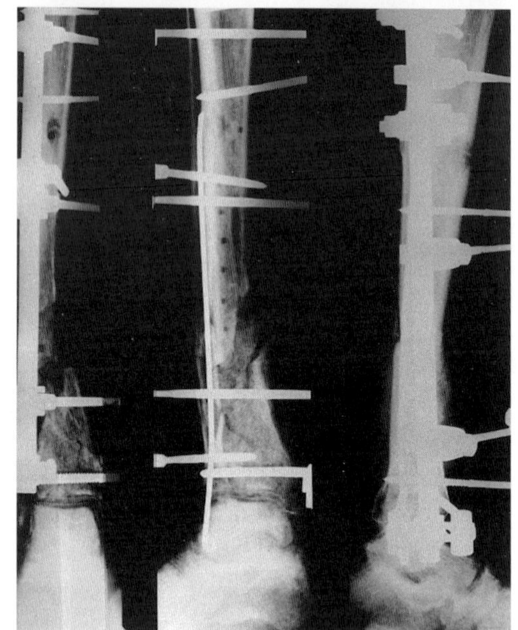

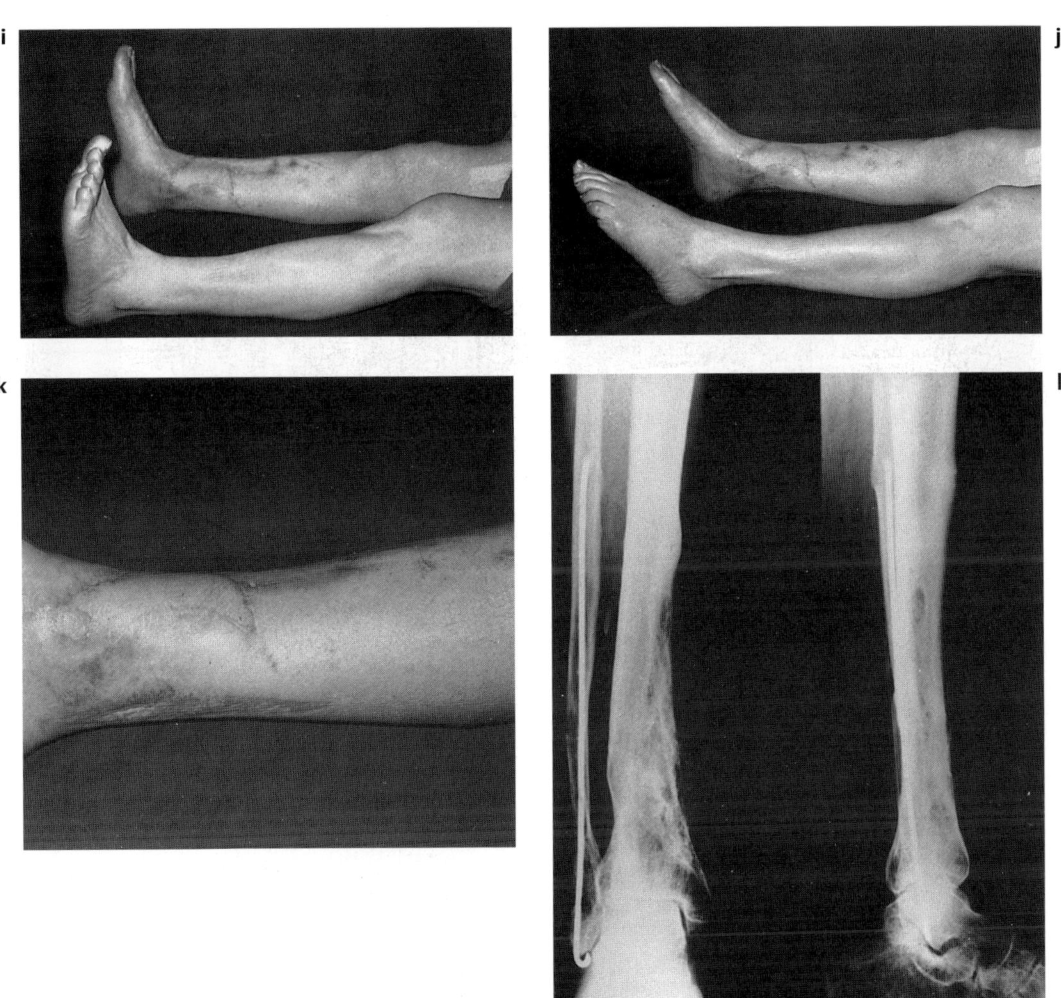

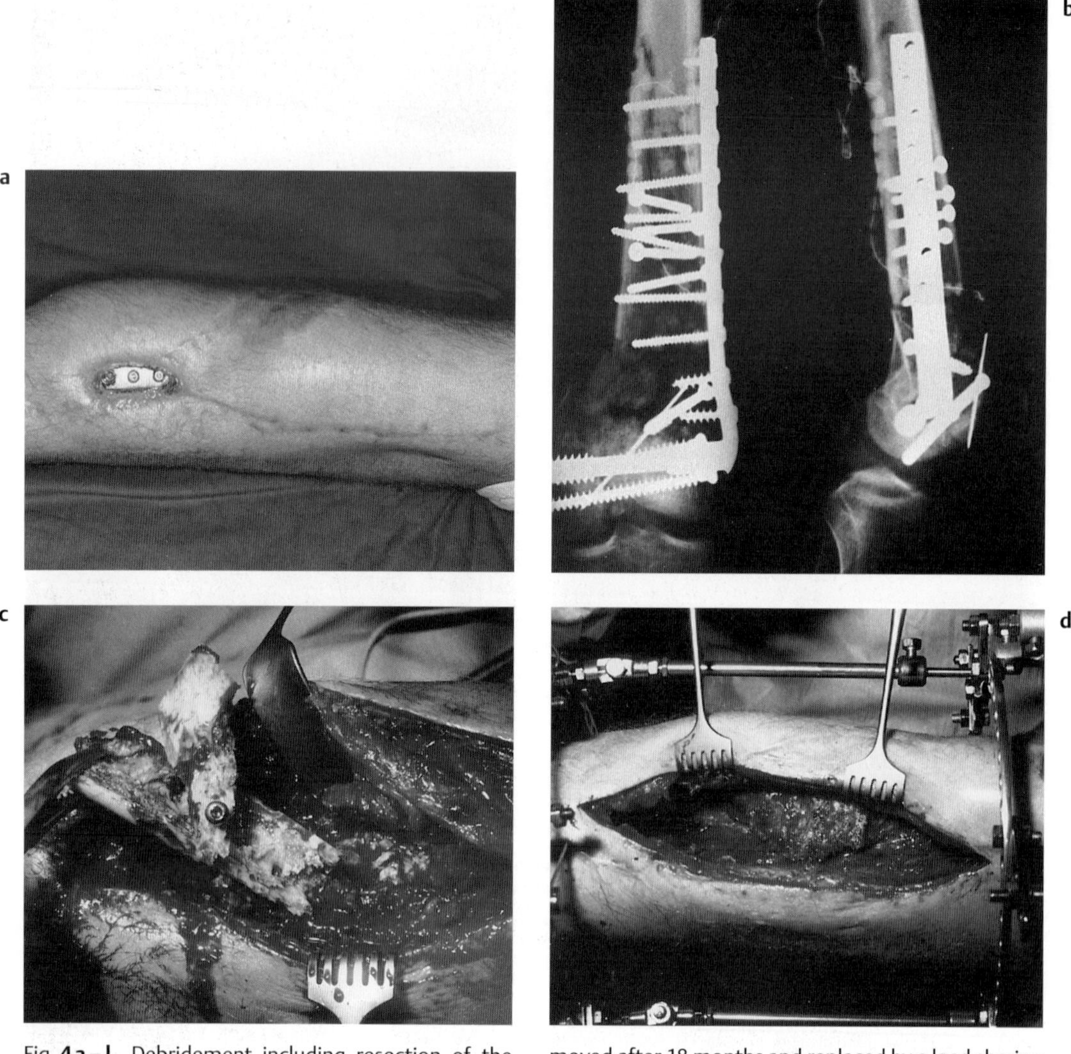

Fig. **4a – l** Debridement including resection of the whole knee led to a defect measuring 20 cm. Stabilization with a ring fixator. A proximal osteotomy and callus distraction via two pulley wires. The fixator was removed after 18 months and replaced by a load sharing orthosis. Full weight bearing was allowed after 8 months. Unstable docking site.

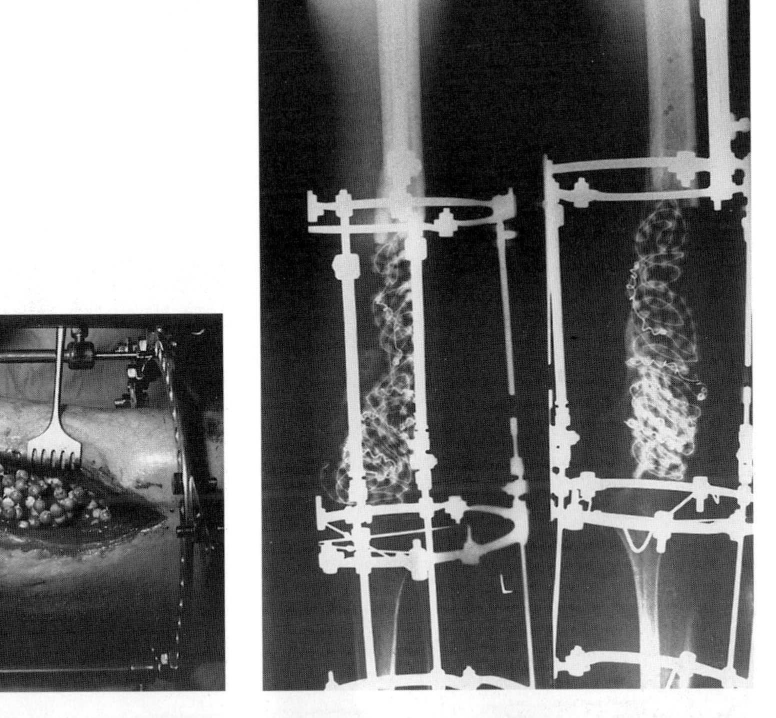

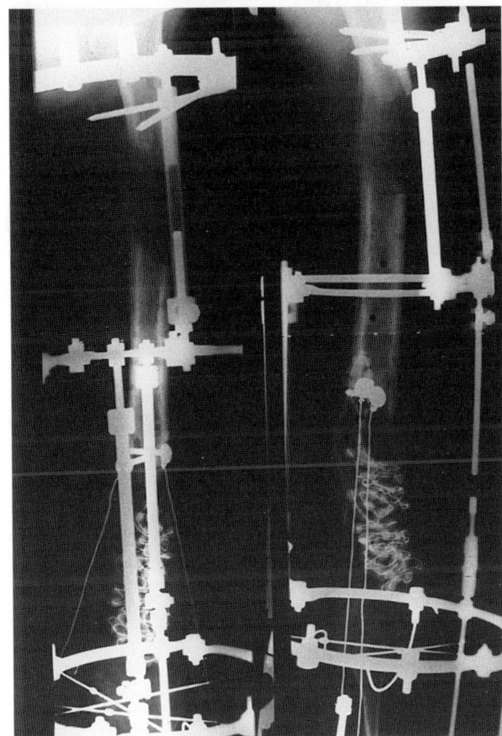

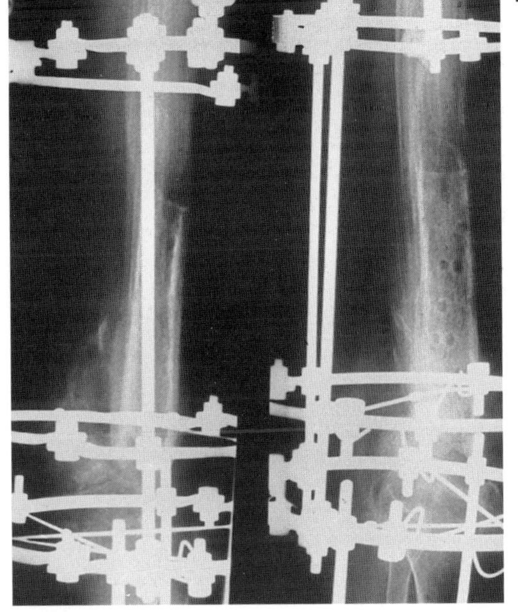

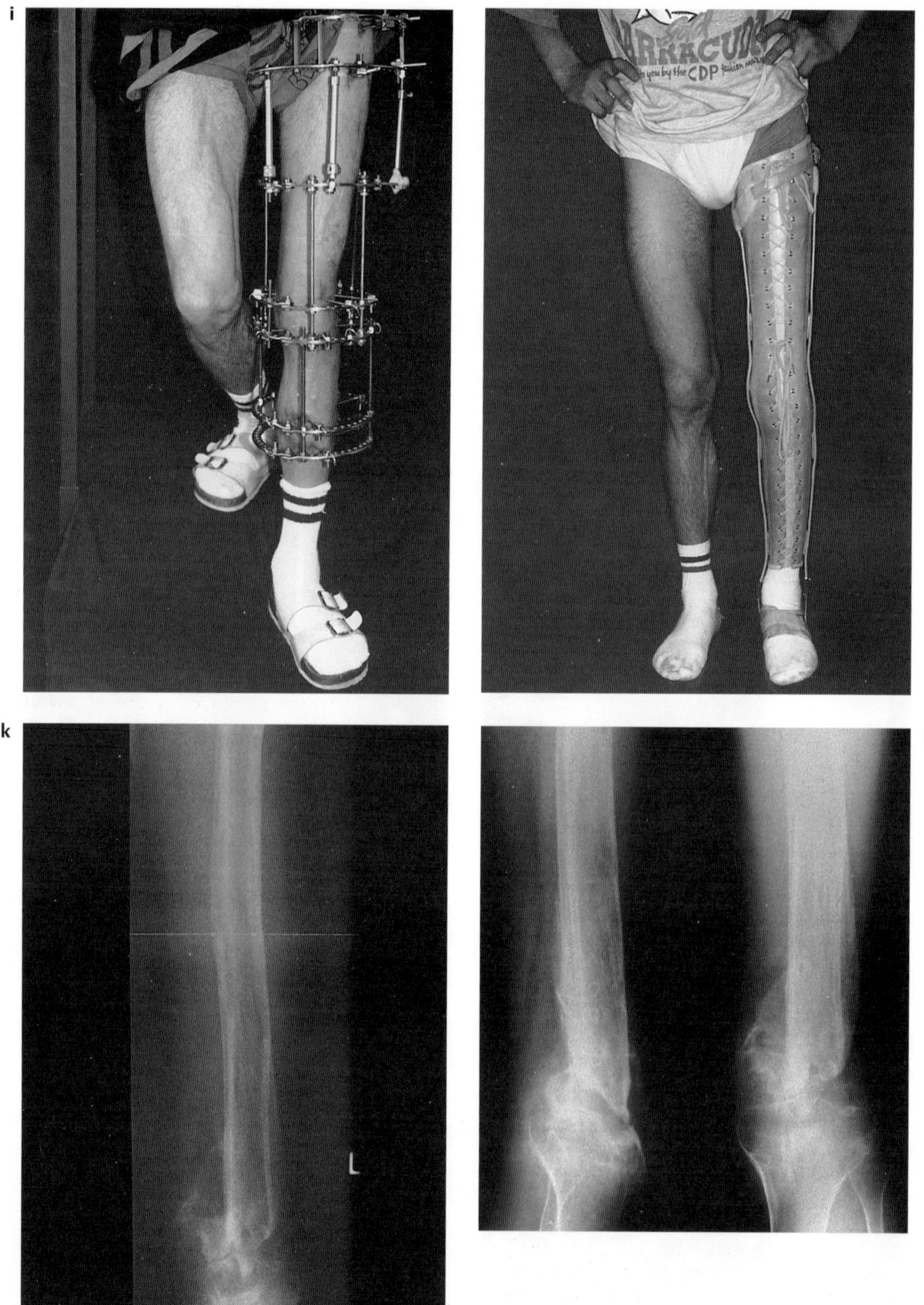

Site	n	Instability	%	Soft tissue defect	%
Femur	158	62	39.2	10	6.4
Tibia	385	217	56.4	166	43.0
Foot	28	–	–	16	57.0
Total	571	279	48.9	192	33.6

Table **1a** Bone infections involving the lower extremity treated between 1976 and 1986

Site	Available for follow-up	Stable without fistula	%	Instability or fistula	Amputation
Femur	155	148	95.5	6	–
Tibia	381	359	94.2	9	13
Foot	28	25	89.3	3	–
Total	564	532	94.3	18	13

Table **1b** Long-term results following bone infections of the lower extremity (1976 – 1986)

tral fixator, Septopal beads were implanted, and a wound closure was obtained with the help of Epigard®. Four weeks later, the first bone graft followed as well as the soft-tissue reconstruction utilizing two sequentially anastomosed free radial flaps, which was carried out by our plastic surgeons. The bone reconstruction required three bone grafts. The function of the upper ankle joint was partially spared. This young man was able to bear full weight 18 months later in an orthopedic shoe and returned to full time employment. The other patient presented with an infection of the distal tibia and talus, as well as with an infectious arthritis of the upper and lower ankle joint. The necrectomy led to a defect of 15 cm and a resection of the hindfoot so that only the calcaneus remained. A large tissue defect was also present. The stabilization was reached with an Ilisarow ring fixator and the soft-tissue defect, which was primarily covered with Epigard®, was reconstructed secondarily with a free latissimus flap three weeks later. At this time, the callus distraction, which required 200 days, was begun. The fixator remained in place for 14 months, the newly formed bone in the distraction area was stable, while the docking site between distal tibia and calcaneus remained unstable, requiring further surgery.

Results and Conclusions

Our large patient population has been studied extensively. In the following a few representative, cumulative numbers are presented. The results of our treatment of osteomyelitis from 1976 until 1986 are shown in Table **1a + b**. During these ten years, a total of 571 infections were treated. To better describe the population dealt with, the rate of instability and soft-tissue defects greater than 6 cm seen in our hospital are depicted. Almost 50% of the patients were cases of pseudarthrosis, defect fractures, and defect pseudarthrosis. One third of the clientele presented with additional soft-tissue defects, especially in the region of the lower leg and foot. A total of 564 of these 571 patients were available for follow-up in 1988, the infection had resolved in 94.3% of the cases (Table **1b**). Only 13 patients had to undergo an amputation, while one patient died while suffering from a still active infection of the femur.

The review of patients with infectious arthritis during the same time frame showed that 163 joint infections of the lower extremity, including one patient with an empyema of the sacroiliac joint, were treated (Table **2a + b**). One-third of the patients had developed a soft-tissue defect larger than six centimeters in diameter as a sign

Table **2a** Joint infections involving the lower extremity treated between 1976 and 1986

Site	n	Soft tissue defect	%
Sacroiliac/hip	30	3	10.0
Knee	47	13	26.5
Ankle	52	25	48.1
Foot	34	12	35.3
Total	163	53	32.5

Site	Available for follow-up	Without fistula	%	With fistula	Amputation
Sacroiliac/hip	30	26	86.7	4	–
Knee	47	45	95.7	1	1
Ankle	52	49	94.2	1	2
Foot	34	29	85.3	3	2
Total	163	149	91.4	9	5

Table **2b**   Long-term results following joint infections of the lower extremity (1976 – 1986)

of the chronicity of the ailment. At the time of the follow-up examination, 91.4% of the infectious processes had been resolved. In only three percent of the cases did the infectious arthritis lead to an amputation – an exceptionally low rate.

Obviously, the resolution of an infection is not always equal to good function – a vital parameter for the affected joint. During the evaluation period from 1982 until 1992, a total of 63 isolated joint infections were treated in our unit. The upper extremity was involved only eight times, while the lower extremity (sacroiliac joint 1; knee 50, ankle 4 instances) was affected in the majority of the cases. Only 26 of the joint infections treated in our hospital had been active for less than 2 weeks. Almost two-thirds of the infections had existed for more than 14 days (between 15 – 28 days: 11 cases; 29 – 180 days: 26 cases). In this population, 30 patients presented with extensive or total destruction of the cartilage. Due to this constellation, only two of these chronic infections were managed arthroscopically, while 55 times the two-step revision described above was carried out. In 6 instances a primary arthrodesis had to be performed. The two-step protocol was successful 96.4% of the time, even though it had to be repeated in some instances. At the time of the follow-up examination, on average 6 years later, in 54 instances or in 85% of this group, the joint was preserved. A total of 9 arthrodeses had to be carried out. The range of motion of the affected joint was on average 70% of the healthy, opposite side.

Finally, we would like to present data from a questionnaire sent to our patients with bone and joint infections treated during the time period from 1979 until 1989. A total of 987 infections of 938 patients with a follow-up of five to fifteen years were evaluated. A total of 68% of the questionnaires were returned, 7.6% of the patients were already decreased, while 24.4% of the patients were lost to follow-up. Of these patients,

41.1% had originally presented with an infection in light of stable bone conditions, 35.6% had infections as well as unstable situation, frequently with a bone defect, while 23.2% suffered from joint infections. In reviewing the data, 80.7% of the patients with primary stability remained infection-free, while 89.7% of the patients, who originally had an unstable situation, did not suffer a recurrence. 80.9% of the joint infections were resolved in the course of treatment. In total, our treatment regimen was successful in 84% of the cases. We view this result to be acceptable, but improvements, especially in the problematic cases are necessary – so further changes in our treatment protocol are to be expected.

We hope that we were able to show that acceptable results can be achieved with a comprehensive and aggressive treatment regimen for infections seen in a trauma clientele.

3

Mineral Biomaterials

New Developments in Implant Coatings: Biomimetics and Tissue Engineering

J. D. de Bruijn, C. A. van Blitterswijk

Introduction

In the past 10 years, abundant research has been performed to obtain, characterize, and optimize plasma-sprayed hydroxyapatite coatings. Such coatings are produced on metallic implants at temperatures of roughly 10,000 °C and are mechanically bound to the substrate. Although it was initially thought that plasma-sprayed hydroxyapatite coatings should be highly crystalline to limit degradation, recent research has indicated that less crystalline, or amorphous coatings are more beneficial from mechanical (Clemens, 1995) and biological (de Bruijn et al., 1992; 1994) points of view. Mechanically, using a rotating beam test under wet conditions (Clemens, 1995), it was shown that amorphous hydroxyapatite coatings were more stable than highly crystalline hydroxyapatite coatings which revealed abundant delamination. Biologically, amorphous hydroxyapatite coatings were shown to bind to bone through a surface apatite layer (de Bruijn et al., 1992; 1994; van Blitterswijk et al., 1993), while more bone apposition was apparent at shorter implantation times, as compared to highly crystalline hydroxyapatite coatings (unpublished results). Irrespective of their crystallinity, some mainly **theoretical** drawbacks of plasma-sprayed hydroxyapatite coatings have been postulated: Bloebaum et al. (1993, 1994) expressed their concern about possible "particulate disease" or bone resorption, as a result of detached hydroxyapatite particles from the plasma-spray coating. This could occur both with highly crystalline coatings that delaminate, or with only partially amorphous coatings that, due to their composition of an amorphous phase alternated by larger crystalline domains (de Bruijn, 1993), can release particles during degradation of the amorphous phase. While we have never observed any disadvantageous biological reactions as a result of loosened hydroxyapatite particles, we do realise that improvements in bioactive coatings

can be made, if not with the attachment of the coating to the substrate, then with a more uniform coating composition, faster bone-bonding properties and osteoinductive capacities.

For such improved, or novel bioactive coatings, several approaches can be pursued. First of all, biomimetics can be used to apply calcium phosphate coatings (Kokubo, 1992). These coatings are produced as a result of incubation of implant materials, in the presence of bioactive glass granules, in so-called simulated body fluids. These fluids mimic human serum in inorganic ion composition and the resulting coating is composed of carbonate apatite crystals, similar to those present in bone, hence the name "biomimetic". Besides similarities to bone apatite crystals, the coating exhibits similarities to the surface carbonate-apatite layer through which bioactive materials bond to bone. Miyaji et al. (1994) have described a way to induce the bioactivity of titanium by means of a chemical treatment with alkaline solutions. This induced bioactivity was indicated by the potential of the chemically treated metal to form a surface carbonate-apatite layer. Herein we strive to produce specific, sub-micron surface structures that can act as nucleation sites for apatite crystal formation. An analogy for this approach was deduced from the fact that water pipes mainly "calcify" at sites where scratches are present (de Groot, 1995). Concurrent with the biomimetic coating process, osteoinductive proteins and growth factors might be co-precipitated to produce not only osteoconductive, but also osteoinductive coatings. The second, more biologically directed approach to obtain bioactive coatings, utilizes so-called bone tissue engineering. With this technique, we strive to coat implants with a layer of patient-own bone tissue *prior* to implantation in the body. For such an approach, mesenchymal cells are isolated via a bone marrow biopsy and grown under specific culture conditions to obtain large quantities of osteogenic cells. These cells are subsequently transferred to the implant material, where they are triggered to start forming bone tissue. When enough bone tissue is produced on the implant materials, they are implanted in the patient, where they are expected to give rise to enhanced bone healing. The concept of growing bone tissue *in vitro* has been widely proven (Davies et al., 1991; de Bruijn et al., 1992; 1996), which indicates the potential of this approach. Herein, we will examine the osteoinductive capacities of *in vitro* produced rat bone tissue by implanting porous hydroxyapatite discs, coated with a bone-like matrix, subcutaneously in syngeneic rats. Resulting ectopic bone formation will prove the osteoinductive capacities of *in vitro* cultured bone-like tissue.

Summarized, the aim of this study is to examine the possible use of a biomimetical approach and a bone-tissue engineering approach to develop new, improved implant coatings.

Materials and Methods

Biomimetic Coatings

Plates of Ti6 A14 V and TiA12.5 Fe were ground using silicon carbide sandpaper and polished with diamond paste to obtain specific surface structure. Other samples of cp-titanium and Ti6 A14 V were etched with a mixture of acidic (HCl and H_2SO_4) and alkaline (NaOH) chemicals respectively, to obtain specific surface structures. All samples were subsequently ultrasonically cleaned in 90% ethanol and rinsed in distilled water. After drying, they were immersed in "calcifying" solutions, such as Hanks Balanced Salt Solution (HBSS), for up to 14 days at 37°C (Leitao et al., 1995). The solution was refreshed every 48 hours and stored at 4°C for the determination of calcium and phosphorus by atomic absorption spectroscopy (AAS) and spectroscopy. The pH of the solution was recorded as a function of time as well as before and after immersion, the surfaces of the samples were examined by scanning electron microscopy (SEM), thin film X-ray diffractometry (XRD), X-ray microanalysis (XRMA), and X-ray photoelectron spectroscopy (XPS).

Bone Tissue Engineering

Bone-matrix culture: Rat bone marrow cells were obtained from the femora of 100–120 gram young adult male albino Fischer rats. The femora were removed and washed 3 times in α-

Minimal Essential Medium (α-MEM-RNA/DNA, Gibco) containing antibiotics in a 10 times higher concentration than usual (see below). After removal of the epiphyses, the bone marrow was flushed out with 6 ml fully supplemented medium per femur (see below). The bone marrow obtained was pooled, so that a uniform cell population was obtained for each experiment. A volume of 0.6 ml cell suspension was seeded onto 2 mm thick macro-porous hydroxyapatite discs with a diameter of about 8 mm, an average pore size of 400 μm and an average void in volume of approximately 30%. Thermanox[tm] coverslips, which served as a control to monitor the progress of the cultures, were seeded with a similar volume of cell suspension. The cultures were maintained in fully supplemented medium, that consisted of α-MEM supplemented with 15% fetal calf serum (FCS, Gibco), 0.1 mg/ml penicillin G (Boehringer-Mannheim), 50 μg/ml gentamicin (Gibco), 0.3 μg/ml fungizone (Gibco), and freshly-added 10^{-8} M dexamethasone (Sigma), 10 mM β-glycerophosphate (Gibco), and 50 μg/ml ascorbic acid (Gibco). The cultures were incubated in a humidified atmosphere of 90% air, 10% CO_2 at 37°C. The medium was changed after the first 24 hours to remove non-adherent cells and was further refreshed three times weekly. During the culturing period, 3 or 4 hydroxyapatite discs were placed in each well of a 6-well plate. As a control, hydroxyapatite discs were placed in cell-free, fully supplemented culture medium in order to examine possible medium-mediated alterations of the samples.

Implantation procedure: After four weeks of culture, control samples and implants with cultured bone matrix were subcutaneously implanted in the back of 7-weeks-old male albino Fischer rats (approximately 250–300 gram). The rats were anesthetised by an intramuscular injection with 0.1 ml Hypnorm per 100 g body weight. The skin was shaved and cleaned with 10% ethanol/iodine and 2 subcutaneous pockets were created on each lateral site of the spine of the back of the rat. One implant was inserted in every pocket resulting in a maximum of 4 subcutaneous implants per rat. For an *in vivo* survival period of 1 week, 5 hydroxyapatite samples with cultured bone matrix and 4 control samples were implanted, while for a survival period of 4 weeks, respectively 6 and 5 samples were implanted.

Light Microscopy

After 1 and 4 weeks the rats were terminated in a CO_2-incubator, followed by cervical dislocation. The samples, with surrounding subcutaneous tissues, were removed and fixed in 1.5 % glutaraldehyde in 0.14 M cacodylate buffer for at least 24 hours at 4 °C. They were subsequently dehydrated through a graded series of alcohol and embedded in methyl methacrylate (MMA). Histological sections, with a thickness of approximately 10 µm, were cut with a modified innerlock diamond saw and stained with methylene blue and basic fuchsin.

Scanning Electron Microscopy

All biological samples were fixed and dehydrated according to the light microscopy procedure and critical point dried from carbon dioxide in a Balzers model CPD 030 Critical Point Dryer. Overlying cell layers were removed with adhesive tape to facilitate examination of the elaborated mineralized extracellular matrix and some samples were freeze fractured in liquid nitrogen to study the bone-biomaterial interface and bone/tissue ingrowth in the pores.

Biomimetic samples were rinsed in double distilled water and dried at 40 °C. All samples were sputter coated with gold or carbon (Balzers sputter coater model SCD 004 in combination with Balzers Carbon evaporation supply model CEA 030), and examined in a Philips S 525 scanning electron microscope at an accelerating voltage of 15 kV, with an attached X-ray microanalysis system (Voyager 700 P118 929).

Results

Biomimetic Coatings

After immersion of the polished samples in HBSS, an increase in pH from 7.5 to approximately pH 8.6 was apparent towards day 7, followed by a drop in pH to approximately pH 8.2. The control HBSS solution, however, maintained a pH of approximately 8.6 (Fig. 1). In correspondence with the drop in pH, both atomic absorption spectrometry and spectrophotometry revealed an increased calcium and phosphorus uptake by the metals. This was attributed to the growth of apatite nuclei on the surfaces of the samples, which was confirmed with scanning electron microscopy. The resulting biomimetic calcium phosphate coating was composed of small needle and

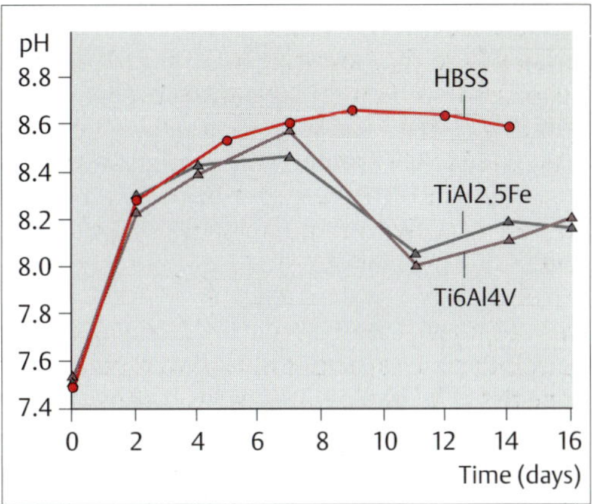

Fig. 1   Graph showing the pH changes as a function of time in a control (●) Hanks Balanced Salt Solution (HBSS), and HBSS in which Ti6 A14 V (▲) and TiA12.5 Fe (▲) samples have been incubated. Incubation of the metallic samples results in a drop of pH around day 7, which corresponds with the formation of a biomimetic calcium phosphate layer.

plate-like crystallites. X-ray microanalysis and X-ray photoelectron spectroscopy confirmed the presence of calcium and phosphorus only after the metals had been immersed in HBSS. The formed coating was identified with thin-film X-ray diffractometry as amorphous with an apatitic structure.

Immersion of the chemically surface-modified samples in calcifying solutions revealed that the formation rate of the surface apatite layer largely depended on the concentration of calcium and phosphate ions present in the solutions. A rapid formation of the biomimetic coating was obtained with higher calcium and phosphate concentrations, and resulted in a mixture of octacalcium phosphate and apatite, while a more gradually formed coating (growth rate of 1 to 3 µm per week) mainly consisted of carbonate apatite (Fig. 2). The latter coating also appeared to be denser in structure when examined with scanning electron microscopy (Fig. 3). Recent experiments have shown that proteins can be co-precipitated during the formation of the biomimetic calcium phosphate coating (Wen, 1997). This possibility provides a good opportunity to coprecipitate growth factors or osteoinductive proteins that could be gradually released during degradation or resorption of the coating. Such experiments are currently being conducted in our laboratory.

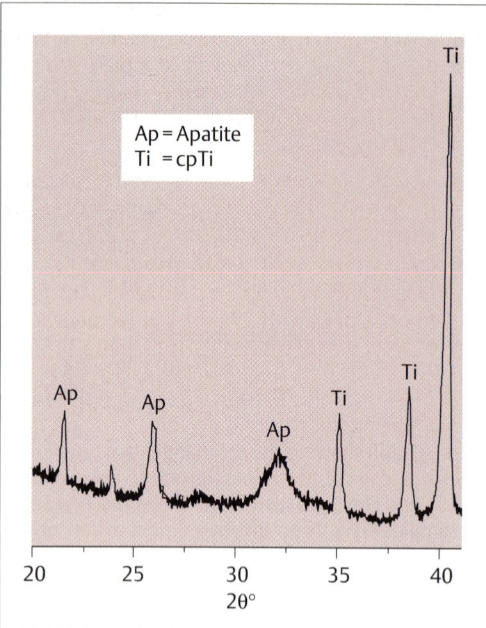

Fig. **2** Thin film X-ray diffractogram of a dense biomimetic calcium phosphate coating deposited by immersion in HBSS for 1 week, which reveals that the coating is composed of apatite (Ap) crystals.

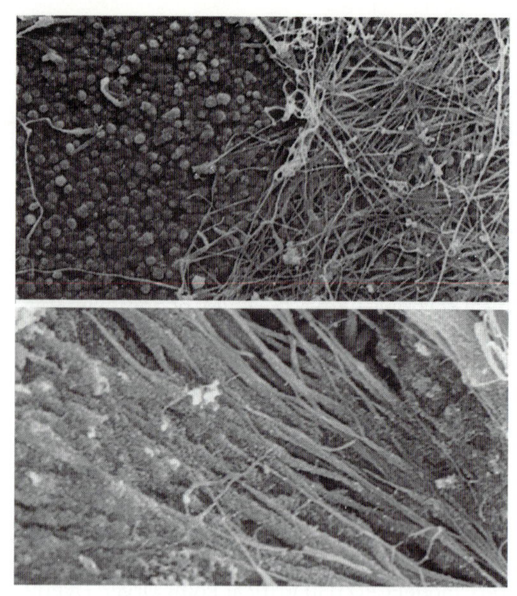

Fig. **4** Scanning electron micrographs showing a cementing layer of afibrillar globules with which the overlying collagenous extracellular matrix is closely associated (**a**). At a high magnification, mineralized collagen fibers can clearly be seen merging to form a bone-like mineralized extracellular matrix (**b**).

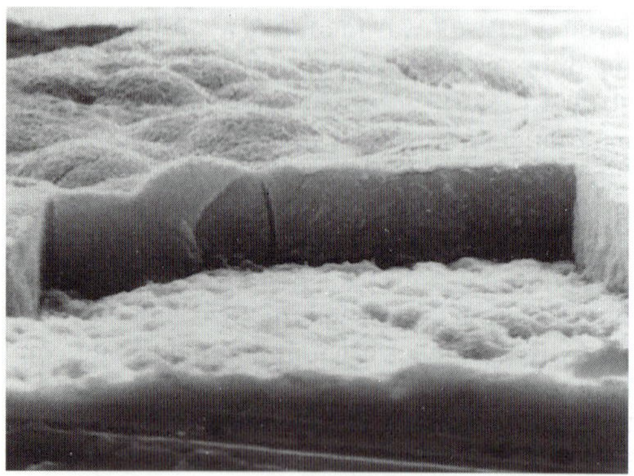

Fig. **3** Scanning electron micrograph of a dense biomimetic calcium phosphate coating precipitated on cp-Ti after 1 week of immersion in HBSS.

Bone Tissue Engineering

Bone-matrix culture: Light microscopy of control bone marrow cell cultures on Thermanox™ showed confluency of the cell layer after 5 to 6 days and nodules were observed after 7 days. Mineralization of the extracellular matrix was light microscopically observed from 2 weeks onward and was only associated with nodules. Scanning electron microscopy revealed the presence of afibrillar globules, which were closely associated with mineralized collagen fibers (Fig. **4**). None of the control hydroxyapatite samples (hydroxyapatite without bone marrow cells) showed mineralized matrix formation. In contrast, the samples combined with marrow cells already revealed new bone formation after 1 week of culture. Bone formation was restricted to the more peripheral pores and the surface of the hydroxyapatite discs, while more central orientated pores hardly contained cultured cells. It seemed that osteoblast layers with extracellular matrix had bridged the pores, instead of following the surface, although this could also be partially attributed to a dehydration artefact. The total amount of mineralized bone-like matrix increased with longer culturing periods (5 and 8 weeks), but was still limited to the periphery of the samples. Although an osteoblast layer and osteoid could not easily be detected, osteocyte-like cells, fully surrounded by a mineralized extracellular matrix, could be seen. The cultured bone-like matrix had a thickness of up to approximately 50 µm.

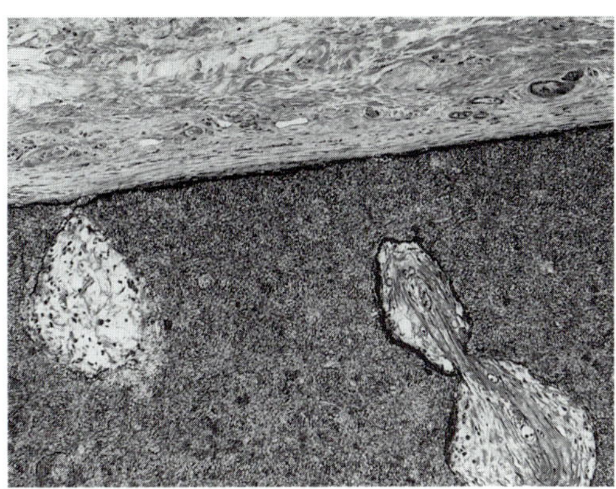

Fig. 5 Light micrograph showing fibrous ingrowth and encapsulation of a control porous hydroxyapatite implant that has been subcutaneously implanted for 4 weeks in a Fischer rat. This indicates and confirms that hydroxyapatite alone does not exhibit osteoinductive properties. Also note the high density of the hydroxyapatite implant, which would be far from optimal with regard to bone-tissue engineering.

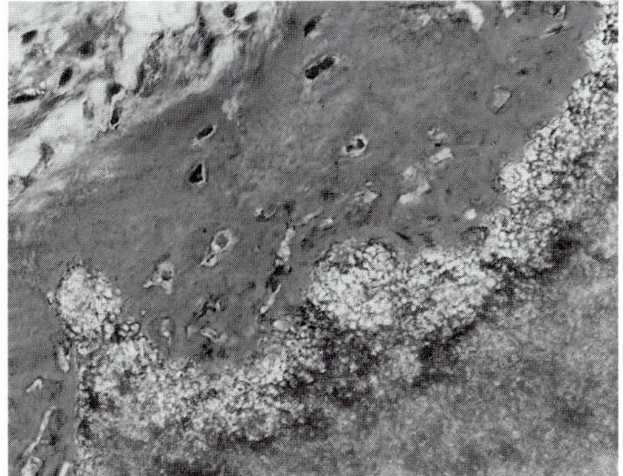

Fig. 6 Light micrograph of bone formation in porous hydroxyapatite that has been subcutaneously implanted for 4 weeks in a Fischer rat, after syngeneic rat bone marrow cells had been cultured in the implant for 4 weeks. Note the newly formed (*de novo*) bone, which is more organised than the mineralized tissue that was formed *in vitro* (not shown). This indicates the *in vivo* osteogenic potential of the bone marrow cell culture system and its potential for bone tissue engineering purposes.

Implantation of hydroxyapatite samples: None of the implanted samples showed microscopic signs of infection or inflammation and fibrous tissue invasion with vascularization into the pore regions could be seen. Limited degradation of the hydroxyapatite surface was apparent both after 8 weeks *in vitro* and after 4 weeks *in vivo*. Although none of the control samples showed bone formation at any of the time periods examined (Fig. 5), newly formed (*de novo*) bone was already apparent 1 week post-operatively in hydroxyapatite samples on which a bone-like matrix had been cultured. This newly formed bone was mainly detected at the periphery of the samples and in the peripheral pores, while the amount of bone tissue increased with time. Four weeks post-operatively, the newly formed bone was organized in structure and exhibited many osteocytes and a peripheral osteoid layer and osteoblast seam (Fig. 6). Although not all pores were filled with bone tissue, it was also observed in more central orientated pores.

Discussion

The results presented herein confirm the potential of both biomimetics and bone-tissue engineering to obtain new implant coatings that can be used for a variety of clinical applications. By using biomimetics, coatings can be produced that are not only more similar to the inorganic component of bone but that are also strongly bound to the metallic implant surface. Although standardized scratch tests have not been performed yet, we have indications that the coating is strongly and seemingly chemically bound to the metallic surface (unpublished results). Another possibility to improve such a coating is to concurrently coprecipitate osteoinductive proteins during the coating process. Maintaining protein activity is feasible due to the fact that biomimetic coatings are produced at temperatures of up to 37 °C.

Theoretically, such a coprecipitation will result in a slow release of osteoinductive material that provides significantly better long-term results than the current procedures. In these procedures, materials are loaded with osteoinductive proteins by incubation in a proteinaceous solution, that will give rise to a burst release shortly after implantation.

In a feasibility study (unpublished), we have been able to coprecipitate bovine serum albumin (BSA) in a biomimetic calcium phosphate coating, which shows the potential of this approach.

The bone tissue engineering approach is a more sophisticated means of obtaining a biological coating on an implant. The results presented herein show that *in vitro* produced bone-like matrix is osteoinductive when implanted *in vivo*. Although it is not yet known what has actually initiated the ectopic bone formation; the mineralized extracellular matrix, the cultured cells, or both, we have clearly shown the potential of this system.

Yoshikawa et al. (1996) have recently reported the osteogenic ability of cultured marrow stromal cells in porous hydroxyapatite after implantation *in vivo*. However, they placed emphasis on the cultured cells by saying that marrow cell-mediated bone formation at ectopic sites (subcutaneously) was seen, but did not mention the possibility of transplanting cultured bone, instead of only osteogenic cells. Our approach therefore significantly differs from theirs. Besides using bone tissue engineering as a coating on implants, it could also be used in porous bone fillers. The advantages of tissue engineered, patient-own bone are many-fold; (I) it is derived from the donor, who only had to donate some bone marrow in order to be able to culture his/her bone tissue, (II) the transfer of, e.g., viruses, is minimal, and (III) the tissue is not only osteoconductive, but also osteoinductive which means that larger defects can be treated. We are currently in the process of fine-tuning the bone culture process for larger mammals (goats, humans), after which we intend to perform *in vivo* experiments in goats.

Conclusions

The reported results indicate that developments such as biomimetics and bone-tissue engineering are promising to obtain a new generation of bioactive and possibly osteoinductive implant coatings.

Acknowledgements

The authors thank Robert Dekker, Wen Bui, Dr. Eugenia Leitao, Yvonne Bovell, Ineke van den Brink, Remco Dalmeijer, and Henk Leenders for their technical help.

References

Bloebaum RD, DuPont JA. Osteolysis from a press-fit hydroxyapatite-coated implant. J Arthroplasty 1993; 8 (2): 195–202.

Bloebaum RD, Beeks D, Dorr LD, Savory CG, DuPont JA, Hofmann AA. Complications with hydroxyapatite particulate separation in total hip arthroplasty. Clinical Orthopaedics 1994; 298: 19–26.

Clemens JAM. Fluorapatite coatings for the osseointegration of orthopaedic implants. Thesis, Leiden University, 1995.

Davies JE, Ottensmeyer P, Shen X, Peel SAF. Early extracellular matrix synthesis by bone cells. In: Davies JE (ed.). The Bone-Biomaterial Interface. University of Toronto Press, Toronto 1991: pp. 214–28.

de Bruijn JD, Davies JE, Klein CPAT, de Groot K, van Blitterswijk CA. Biological response to calcium phosphate ceramics. In: Ducheyne P, et al. (eds.). Bone-Bonding Biomaterials. Reed Healthcare Communications, Leiderdorp, The Netherlands 1992: pp. 57–72.

de Bruijn JD. Calcium phosphate biomaterials: bone-bonding and biodegradation properties. Thesis, Leiden University, The Netherlands 1993.

de Bruijn JD, Bovel YP, Klein CPAT, de Groot K, van Blitterswijk CA. Structural arrangements at the interface between plasma sprayed calcium phosphates and bone tissue *in vivo*. Biomaterials 1994; 15 (7): 543–50.

de Bruijn JD, van den Brink I, Bovel YP. Development of a human bone marrow culture to examine the interface between apatite and bone formed *in vitro*. In: Kokubo T, Nakamura T (eds.). Bioceramics, Volume 9. Elsevier Science Ltd., Amsterdam 1996: pp. 45–8.

de Groot K. Personal communication 1995.

Kokubo T. Bioactivity of glasses and glass ceramics. In: Ducheyne, et al. (eds.). Bone-Bonding Biomaterials. Reed Healthcare Communications, Leiderdorp, The Netherlands 1992: 31–46.

Leitao E, Barbosa MA, de Groot K. *In vitro* calcification of orthopaedic implant materials. J Mater Sci Mater Med 1995; 6 (12): 849–52.

Miyaji F, Zhang X, Yao T, Kokubo T, Ohtsuki C, Kitsugi T, Yamamuro T, Nakamura T. Chemical treatment of Ti metal to induce its bioactivity. In: Andersson OH, Yli-Urpo A (eds.). Bioceramics, Volume 7. Butterworth-Heinemann Ltd., London 1994: pp. 119–24.

van Blitterswijk CA, Bovell YP, Flach JS, Leenders H, van den Brink J, de Bruijn JD. Variations in hydroxyapatite crystallinity: Effects on interface reactions. In: Geesink R, et al. (eds.). Hydroxylapatite coatings in orthopaedic surgery. Raven press, New York 1993: pp. 33–47.

Wen HB. Personal communication, 1997.

Yoshikawa T, Ohgushi H, Tamai S. Immediate bone forming capability of prefabricated osteogenic hydroxyapatite. J Biomed Mater Res 1996; 32: 481–92.

Bone Graft Substitutes: Clinical Studies using Coralline Hydroxyapatite

E. C. Shors

Introduction

Reconstructing of defects in or on bone is the cornerstone of orthopedic surgery. Using the patient's own bone from a donor site has traditionally been the standard for bone grafting procedures. This is because autogenous bone is both osteoconductive and osteoinductive. That is, it serves as a physical structure on which new bone can deposit, i.e., osteoconduction, and it provides growth factors that initiate and sustain bone formation, i.e., osteoinduction. In addition, it is not immunogenic or pathogenic. There, nevertheless, remains a critical need for a bone graft substitute for treating defects in bone or for augmenting existing bone. This need is driven by the desire of surgeons and patients to reduce or eliminate the secondary procedure required for harvesting bone directly from the patients ilium or other site. The prevailing rationale for a substitute is its ability to spare patients the morbidity associated with harvesting bone grafts. Clinical studies have shown that the incidence for this morbidity can be as high as 21 % for minor complications and 9 % for major complications (Younger et al., 1989). Major complications include pain for longer than 6 months, infection, dysesthesia, wound drainage, and reoperation. In addition, a bone graft substitute can reduce the operative time, increase the availability of adequate quantities, and can assure consistent quality.

One alternative source to autogenous bone grafting is to use allograft bone. The advantages of allograft bone are that it is osteoconductive and that it has good mechanical properties. Although controversial, it may, if it is from an appropriate donor and processed properly, also have limited osteoinductive properties. These perceived advantages are outweighed in many cases, however, because allograft can induce immunogenicity and pathogenicity. Like autograft, its quality may be inconsistent.

The science of tissue engineering has inspired the concept of using synthetic implants to initiate and promote the patient's own healing response to form new bone. For this concept, a matrix is manufactured and used which causes bone to grow into, when it is placed in a bone defect. This approach was first demonstrated with inert ceramics and metals, such as alumina or titanium. Hydroxyapatite, the mineral content of bone, has been shown to be a superior material because it is osteophillic. That is, bone will grow on to its surface and form a chemical bond to the material (White and Shors, 1986). A requirement for bone formation is that the implant remain in place and resorb very slowly and only after complete bone incorporation. Hydroxyapatite has a slow degradation rate. Calcium carbonate and other calcium sulfates, by contrast, resorb much too rapidly to assure bone incorporation. Ceramics made from the mineral content of bone, i.e., hydroxyapatite, have been shown to be osteoconductive and osteophillic, particularly if they have interconnecting pores. Several studies have shown that the size of the interconnecting pores must be greater than 100 microns to facilitate bone ingrowth (White and Shors, 1986). The challenge for biomaterial engineers has been to synthetically make such a structure.

Coralline hydroxyapatite is a unique porous implant for filling voids in bone or augmenting deficient bone. It serves as a framework for the regeneration of bone. The implant is derived from a proprietary technology which chemically converts the calcium carbonate skeleton of specific marine corals to hydroxyapatite (White and Shors, 1986). The result is a biocompatible, osteoconductive material with interconnected porosity. The interconnected porosity in the coralline hydroxyapatite is similar to the microstructure of natural bone. Coralline hydroxyapatite provides a biocompatible osteoconductive matrix for tissue ingrowth, vascularization, and deposition of new bone.

Since the early 1970's, more than fifty animal studies have been conducted to evaluate Pro Osteon 500 porous hydroxyapatite as a bone void filler (Holmes et al., 1986; Holmes et al., 1987; Martin et al., 1993). Clinical reports have substantiated this result in a variety of applications (Bucholz et al., 1989; Lewonowshi and Dorr, 1994; Wolfe et al., 1995).

The study presented here is from a multi-center, controlled, clinical trial designed to substantiate the safety and efficacy of the Pro Osteon for the repair of fractures in patients. This clinical study clearly indicates the suitability of the Pro Osteon as a bone graft substitute for the repair of fractures.

Methods and Materials

This was a multi-center study conducted at nine research institutions in the United States. The nine centers that participated are the University of Texas, Dallas, the University of California, Davis, University of California, San Diego, University of South Florida, Tampa, University of Rhode Island, Providence, University of Illinois, Chicago, Tahoe Fracture Clinic, Tahoe, California, New York State University, Brooklyn, and the University of California, San Francisco. Patients were enrolled from 1982 through 1988.

Coralline porous hydroxyapatite was provided in block and granular forms. The blocks had an average pore diameter of 500 microns and a porosity of 65%. There were two sizes of the blocks: 15 × 15 × 30 mm and 10 × 20 × 50 mm. The trade name for this implant is Pro Osteon 500 porous hydroxyapatite (Interpore International, Irvine, California). The granular form for this study was made by the same process with a different starting material. The granules had an average pore diameter of 200 microns and a porosity of 50%. The size of the granules was 450–1000 micron in diameter. The trade name for this material was Interpore 200 porous hydroxyapatite (Interpore International, Irvine, California). This material is also called Pro Osteon 200 porous hydroxyapatite. All implants were presterilized by the manufacturer using radiation sterilization.

Reconstruction using the principals of osteoconduction dictated that three requirements be accomplished. Firstly, the implant must be in direct apposition to surrounding bone. This apposition should be within one millimeter at as much of the surface of the implant as possible. Second-

ly, the surrounding bone must be viable. Factors that decrease viability are devascularization, infection and certain metabolic bone diseases. Thirdly, the interface between the surrounding bone and implant must be stabilized. In most cases with large defects for treating fracture, this was accomplished with internal fixation. These three requirements are sometimes called the *"Triad of Osteoconduction"*.

To complete the reconstruction, the blocks were generally shaped by the surgeon to the contours of the defect. The goal of the surgical team was to fill, as completely as possible, the entire defect volume with the porous implant using one or more blocks. Although Pro Osteon blocks were used in all cases, in some cases, the granules were used to fill in the spaces between blocks and between blocks and the surrounding bone. In some cases the defect was shaped to the contours of the implant. This approach helped to assure fulfillment of the requirement for apposition to surrounding bone. It also allows the implant to serve as a biomechanical buttress. This is because the compressive strength is similar to cancellous bone, approximately 3 MPa. Further, this procedure increases the ability to use the block forms of the material, thereby assuring continuity of the reconstruction with the implant and maximizing the incidence and completeness of bone ingrowth.

Profile of Patient Population

Clinical testing of Pro Osteon began in 1982 and included 167 patients with 174 defects enrolled at nine clinical test sites. Over 80% of the study patients had orthopedic defects caused by fractures. The total defect population consisted of the following diagnostic subsets: cyst/tumor (N = 11), delayed union and non-union (N = 26), and acute fractures (N = 137). The acute fractures were subdivided into three groups: short bone fracture (N = 2), diaphyseal fracture (N = 24), and metaphyseal fracture (N = 111).

Statistical analyses were conducted on a metaphyseal subset of the total patient population that had defects filled with Pro Osteon only. There were 81 patients with 82 defects. The subset was analyzed to determine the healing patterns of these patients, and the results were compared to the healing patterns of a control group of patients who were treated concurrently with autogenous bone graft.

The mean age of the 81 patients was 37 years, with males averaging 35 years and females averaging 42 years. The mean length of follow-up exceeds more than 10 years at this time.

The mean defect volume for all defects treated with Pro Osteon was 13 cc. The range was less than one cubic centimeter to a maximum of approximately 250 cc. For most defects with a implant volume of more than 30 cc, autograft was mixed with the implant. For just the metaphyseal defects, the mean defect volume was 8.9 cc with most defect volumes being in the 1 – 20 cc range.

Eighty percent of the defects treated were located in the tibia, both proximal and distal. The remaining defects were in the femur (11%), radius (7%), and other sites (2%). In all but one patient, the severity of the defect was judged by the investigators to be moderate to severe. Fracture types were primarily a combination of comminuted and compression fractures, although pure types were also represented. Pure comminuted fractures represented 34%, pure compressive fractures represented 25%, and combination fractures constituted the remainder (51%). Thirteen of the 82 defects treated were open, 69 were closed. Stabilization was achieved by internal fixation in 79 of the defects.

Outcomes Analysis

To determine the effectiveness of clinical healing, the patients were evaluated for degree of pain at rest, degree of pain during weight bearing, and the status of functional impairment. In addition, radiographs were examined (Figs. 1 and 2). For statistical analysis, the time of radiographic healing was defined as occurring when new bone obscured the fracture lines (Sartoris et al., 1986; Sar-

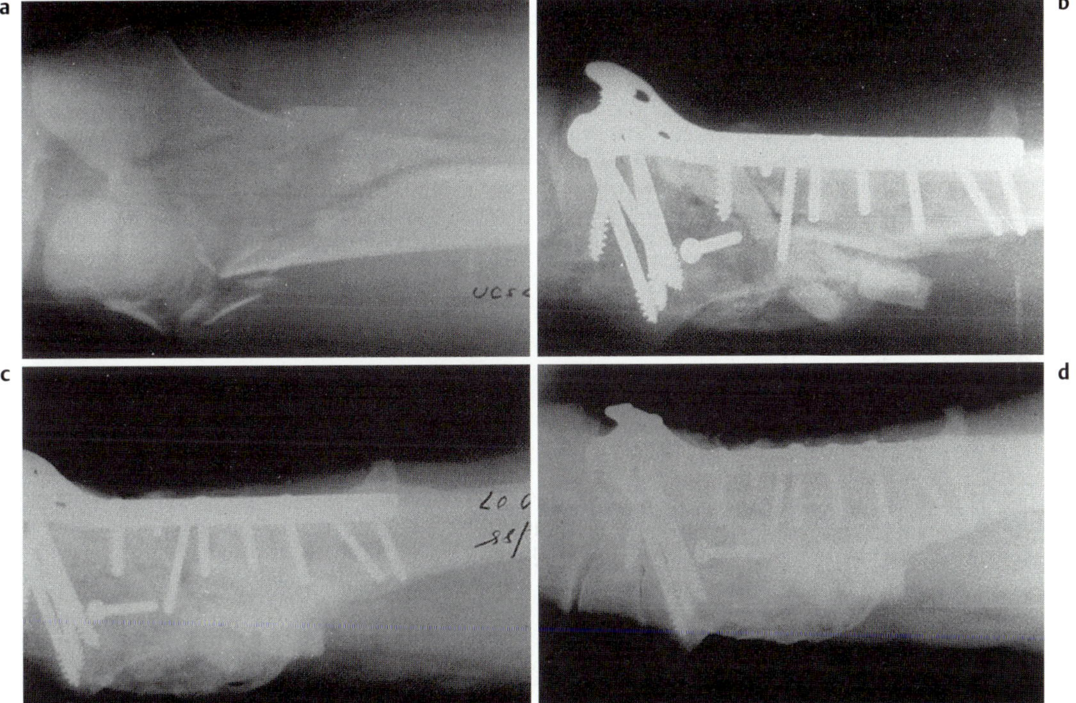

Fig. 1 (a) This patient sustained a femoral fracture involving the distal diaphysis and metaphysis. Preoperative radiograph shows a comminuted fracture. The fracture was reduced with a combination of Pro Osteon blocks and granules. (b) Three-month radiograph shows early consolidation of the callous. The outlines of the blocks are evident but the bone has grown up to the implant. There is no evidence of a radiographic halo. (c) A 10-month radiograph shows further maturation of the fracture. The outlines of the blocks are less discernable, indicating bone incorporation and fracture repair. (d) A 26-month radiograph (04/04/87) shows complete healing. The outlines of the implants are not readily evident. There may be some resorption of the implant.

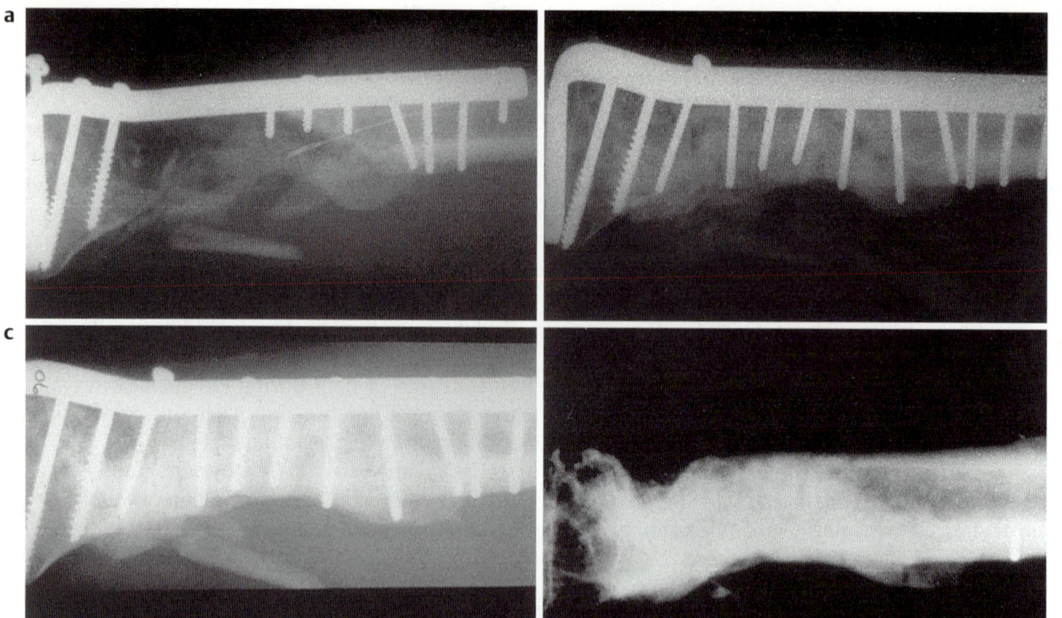

Fig. 2   (**a**) This patient sustained a severe distal femoral diaphyseal fracture while competitively snow skiing. She was reconstructed with ORIF and bone grafting from her iliac crest. Nevertheless, her fracture became a non-infected nonunion which did not resolve with internal electrical bone stimulation. She was then regrafted with Pro Osteon blocks and granules in combination with morselized iliac crest autograft. (**b**) Two months postoperation radiograph indicates reconstruction with Pro Osteon. (**c**) The internal hardware was removed 24 months after reconstruction with Pro Osteon. This radiograph at 37 months shows consolidation of the fracture. Although not recommended by her clinician, the patient returned to competitive level skiing. (**d**) Complete healing is shown after hardware removal by this radiograph at 61 months post reconstruction.

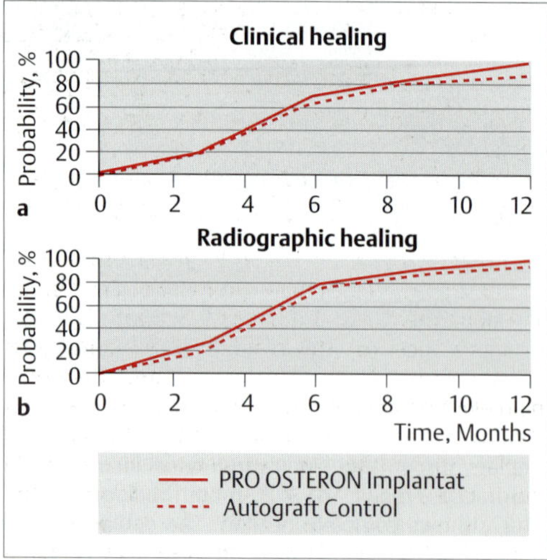

toris et al., 1987). These data were subjected to life table analyses (Fig. **3**). The median time to clinical healing was 4.8 months with the median time to radiographic healing being 4.5 months. Life table analyses indicated that the probability of Pro Osteon treated defects being clinically or radiographically healed at 12 months post-operatively was 94 percent. In three centers, 44

Fig. 3   (**a**) Life table analysis of clinical healing shows that there was no difference in the incidence of clinical healing for patients treated with Pro Osteon or autograft. The mean time for healing of both populations was approximately 4.5 months. (**b**) Life table analysis of radiographic healing shows that, like clinical healing, the rate of healing was not different for patients treated with Pro Osteon or autograft. As judged by the surgeon and independent radiologist, the healing was typically completed at 4.2 months.

concurrent autograft controls were compared to 52 defects in 51 patients receiving Pro Osteon implants. This autogenous control group was also compared to the metaphyseal patient group. Although mathematically the patients with Pro Osteon healed faster than autograft controls, the differences were not statistically different. There was no statistical difference in the probability of radiographic or clinical healing.

Adverse reactions which occurred during the study were similar in type and frequency to those normally seen in surgical procedures involving the use of bone graft and internal fixation. Complications included superficial and deep wound infection, hardware damage, hardware removal, implant removal, delayed or non-union, loss of reduction, amputation, hematoma, wound dehiscence, and osteomyelitis. Reported complications were not caused or exacerbated by the Pro Osteon implant.

A comparison of complication rates was made between patients treated with Pro Osteon and the patients treated with autogenous bone. Twelve month event-free rates for all complica-

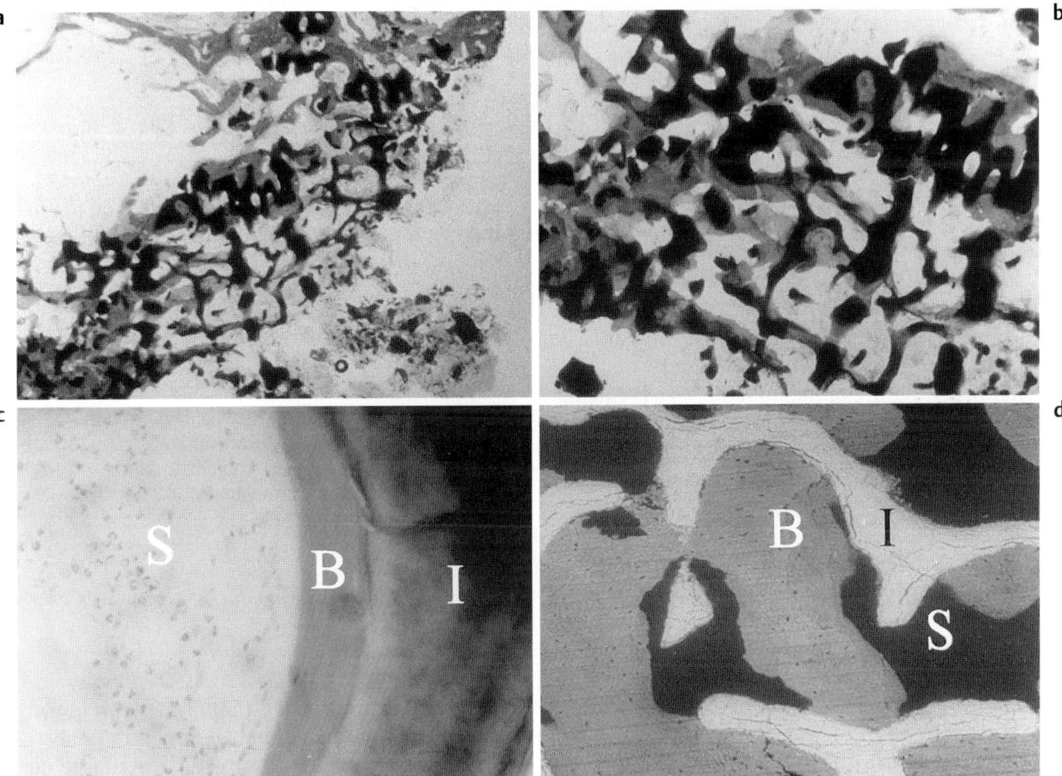

Fig. 4　(a) This low power micrograph from a patient biopsy was obtained using a biopsy needle. It is approximately 2.5 mm in diameter and 8 mm long. The specimen was processed by non-decalcified embedding and stained. The regenerated bone (brownish orange) is evident throughout the pores of Pro Osteon implant. (b) This medium power micrograph from same biopsy shows that the regenerated bone is primarily in direct apposition to the porous hydroxyapatite. This demonstrates the osteoconductive property of Pro Osteon. (c) This high power micrograph from same biopsy illustrates that the regenerated bone (B) is mature lamellar bone and deposited directly onto the internal surface of the implant (I). This demonstrates the osteophillic property of Pro Osteon. The bone marrow and other soft tissue (S) is normal in appearance. (d) This medium power micrograph (40 ×) is from a human biopsy as viewed using scanning electron microscopy with a backscatter electron detector. This method facilitates the histometry. The implant (I) is white, the regenerated bone (B) in the pores is gray, and the soft tissue (S) is black. Note that the technique discriminates the osteocyte lacunae within the bone. This image was then digitized to determine the volume fraction of the components and the surface area of the implant covered by bone.

tions were calculated and compared for significant differences. The results did not show significant differences for any comparisons.

Histology and Histometry of Biopsies

Histological and histometric evaluation of biopsy specimens taken from defects during hardware removal provided a unique opportunity to evaluate the healed implant/bone composite. Thirty-seven biopsy specimens were taken with a median time to biopsy of 15.2 months (range = 7 – 88 months). Thirty-four of the biopsies had bone ingrowth based on conventional stained histology (Fig. 4) and scanning electron microscopy with a back-scatter electron detector SEM-BSE. The method for determining the histometry from SEM-BSE has been described by Holmes et al. (1987). This method has been shown to be free of artifact, operator-independent, and amenable to analysis of large data bases. The method includes the quantification of the volume fractions, as a percentage of three components: implant, bone, and soft tissue. The volume fraction of implant was described as a function of time to determine the resorption rate of the implants. In addition, SEM-BSE can be used to determine the osteophillic nature of the implant. This is calculated by partitioning, as a percentage, the area of the implant covered by either bone or soft tissue. The higher the surface area covered by bone relative to the quantity of bone, the higher is the osteophillic nature of the implant.

Fifteen biopsy specimens were of sufficient size and quality to analyze for volume fraction of bone, implant, and soft tissue. Samples analyzed histometrically (Fig. 5) showed the average volume fraction of new bone in the implant was 39 percent, with the remainder of the volume being occupied by the Pro Osteon implant (31%) and soft tissue (30%). These biopsy data provide direct evidence of the effectiveness of the Pro Osteon as a scaffolding for bony ingrowth with direct contact of bone tissue to the implant surface. Biopsy specimens were also analyzed to determine the rate of degradation of the implant (Fig. 5). Linear regression of volume fraction of implant versus time indicated that the rate of resorption is slow, estimated to be 5 – 10 percent per year, and clinically insignificant in the metaphysis.

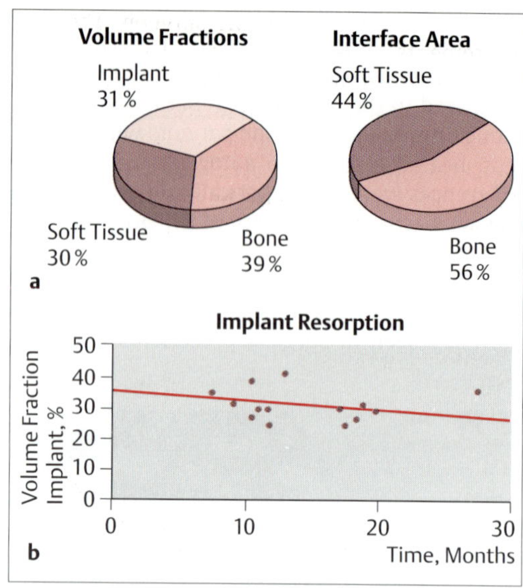

Fig. 5 (a) Histometry was used to partition the patient biopsies into bone, implant, or soft tissue, as percentages (left). The average volume fractions were obtained at approximately 15 months after implantation with Pro Osteon. The histometry also determined the internal surface area of implant covered by bone or soft tissue. Note that this interface area is preferentially covered by bone, demonstrating the osteophillic and osteoconductive properties of the implant. (b) Implant resorption was demonstrated by correlating the volume fraction of implant in biopsies to the time of implantation. The regression line tilts down, indicating slow resorption of the Pro Osteon.

Conclusions

This study demonstrated that Pro Osteon porous hydroxyapatite is an effective bone graft substitute for use in patients to reconstruct large defects in bone after fracture. It substantiated the relevance of the vast pre-clinical animal studies that anticipated this result. From this massive data base, it can be concluded that this material is osteophillic and osteoconductive. When meeting the requirements for osteoconduction, it is an appropriate alternative to autografting, the historical standard for bone grafting procedures. In some cases, it may be superior to autograft because of Pro Osteon's consistent mechanical properties and "off the shelf" availability. To assure a consistent result, it is a obligatory, however, that the three requirements for osteoconduction be achieved by the surgeon. These requirements, called the "Triad of Osteoconduction", are proximity, viability, and stability. To accomplish this, the implant must be in apposition to the surrounding bone, the surrounding bone must be viable, and the entire construct, particularly the interface, must be stabilized. This is achievable in the repair of most acute metaphyseal fractures of long bones. Therefore, Pro Osteon is an appropriate bone graft substitute.

Acknowledgements

I want to offer my sincere appreciation to the clinical investigators whose vital contributions made this study possible. They are Drs. Robert Bucholz and Vert Mooney (University of Texas, Dalla, TX), Dr. Michael Chapman (University of California, Davis, CA), Dr. Wayne Ackeson (University of California, San Diego, CA), Dr. Philip Spiegel (University of South Florida, Tampa, FL), Dr. Thomas Einhorn (State University of New York, Brooklyn, NY), Dr. Peter Trafton (Brown University, Providence, RI), Dr. Keith Swanson (Tahoe Fracture Clinic, Tahoe, CA) and Dr. Lorraine Day (University of California, San Francisco, CA). In addition, I would like to thank Dr. Ralph Holmes (University of California, San Diego) for performing the histology and histometry on the human biopsies.

References

Bucholz RW, Carlton A, Holmes R. Interporous hydroxyapatite as a bone graft substitute in tibial plateau fractures. Clinical Orthopaedics and Related Research 1989; 240: 53 – 62.

Holmes RE, Bucholz RW, Mooney V. Porous hydroxyapatite as a bone graft substitute in diaphyseal defects: A histometric study. Journal of Orthopaedic Research 1987; 5 (1): 114 – 21.

Holmes RE, Bucholz RW, Mooney V. Porous hydroxyapatite as a bone-graft substitute in metaphyseal defects. Journal of Bone and Joint Surgery (Am) 1986; 68 (6): 904 – 11.

Holmes R, Mooney V, Bucholz R, Tencer A. A coralline hydroxyapatite bone graft substitute. Clinical Orthopaedics and Related Research 1984; 188: 252 – 62.

Holmes RE, Hagler HK, Coletta CA. Thick-section histometry of porous hydroxyapatite implants using backscattered electron imaging. Journal of Biomedical Material Research 1987; 21 (6): 731 – 9.

Lewonowski K, Dorr L. Revision of cementless total knee Arthroplasty with massive osteolytic lesions. The Journal of Arthroplasty 1994: 9.

Martin RB, Chapman MW, Sharkey NA, Zissimos SL, Bay B, Shors EC. Bone ingrowth and mechanical properties of coralline hydroxyapatite 1 year after implantation. Biomaterials 1993; 14 (5): 341 – 8.

Sartoris DJ, Gershuni DH, Akeson WH, Holmes RE, Resnick D. Coralline hydroxyapatite bone graft substitutes: preliminary report of radiographic evaluation. Radiology 1986; 159 (1): 133 – 7.

Sartoris DJ, Kusnick C, Resnick D. New concepts in bone grafting. Orthopaedic Review 1987; 3: 153 – 63.

White E, Shors EC. Biomaterial aspects of Interpore 200 porous hydroxyapatite. Dental Clinics of North America 1986; 30 (1): 49 – 57.

Wolfe SW, Easterling KJ, Yoo HH. Arthroscopic-assisted reduction of distal radius fractures. The Journal of Arthroscopic and Related Surgery 1995; 11 (12): 706 – 14.

Younger E, Chapman MW. Morbidity at bone graft donor sites. Journal of Orthopaedic Trauma 1989; 3: 192 – 5.

Zdeblick TA, Cooke ME, Kunz DN, Wilson D, McCabe RP. Anterior cervical discectomy and fusion using a porous hydroxyapatite bone graft substitute. Spine 1994; 19: 2348 – 57.

Bone Substitutes as Drug Carriers

B. Nies

Bone substitute materials are considered as potential drug carriers for the treatment of local bone diseases and for the stimulation of bone regeneration.

Among the most intensively investigated applications are the

- protection of bone implants – especially the bone substitute itself – against foreign body infection,
- prophylaxis and treatment of localized bone infections in combination with surgical intervention, and
- improvement of fracture healing and bone defect filling in orthopedics and traumatology.

Accordingly, antibiotics and bone growth-stimulating drugs are of special interest for the combination with bone substitute materials.

The attractivity of bone substitutes as drug carriers is based on

- their biocompatibility – bioactivity,
- the opportunity to be left *in situ* when antimicrobial treatment is successful,
- the opportunity to preserve or augment autograft, and
- the potential synergistic action in combination with bone growth stimulating drugs.

For the development of bone substitute-drug combinations many open questions remain in spite of the investigational work performed so far.

An evaluation of such important questions for anti-infective drugs and growth factors is summarized in Table **1.**

Whereas for combinations with antibiotics, effective drug release profiles have been evaluated and most technical questions can be solved with existing technology, almost no such solutions are already available for combinations with growth factors. Especially, the questions concerning production and sterilization technology

Table 1 Bone substitute-drug combinations

Typical Problems

Identification and adjustment of a suitable drug
 release profile
Homogeneous drug distribution
Stability of drug-carrier combination
Production – sterilization technology

Solutions Available?

	Anti-infective drugs	Growth factors
Release profile	+	–
Homogeneity	±	±
Stability	+	–
Technology	+	–

will determine the progress of development projects for bone substitutes with incorporated growth factors. Consequently I will focus, therefore, on bone substitutes with antibiotics.

A typical development program includes the following initial steps:

- Identification of the relevant requirements for the selected indication.
- Selection of the appropriate antibiotic (-combination).
- Determination of the optimal antibiotic release profile.
- Adjustment of medical requirements and technical opportunities.

Especially for antibacterial therapy of local bone infections it is necessary to achieve a very high antibacterial activity and an optimized release profile, as it has to be assumed that even after suitable surgical treatment a high bacterial burden will remain in the wound and the surrounding tissue.

In our development of an effective bone substitute-antibiotic combination we selected gentamicin and clindamycin as appropriate drugs since they cover most of the typical bacterial spectrum of chronic osteomyelitis (Fig. **1**).

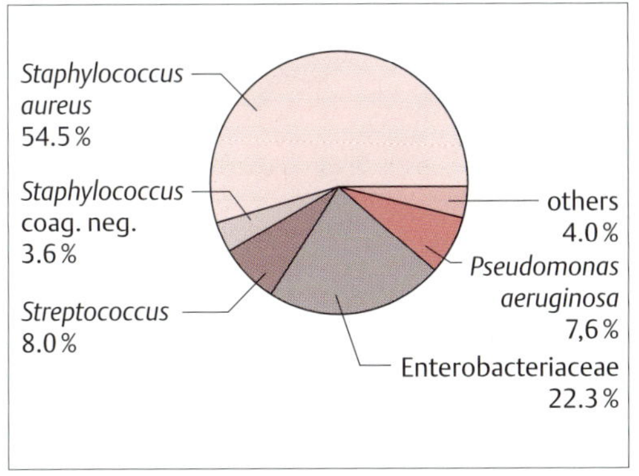

Fig. **1**　Chronic osteomyelitis-bacterial spectrum.

In a series of simulated release kinetic experiments we determined the concentration time curves that most effectively led to a rapid reduction of bacterial count in our *in vitro* model. The example in Figure **2** shows that a modification in the simulated release profile of gentamicin – constant levels of 10 µg/ml versus continuously decreasing levels starting at 100 µg/ml and falling to 10 µg/ml – greatly influences the initial velocity of bacterial killing, even when clindamycin levels are set constant at 10 µg/ml in both runs and when the bacterial strain is susceptible to both drugs.

This optimized drug release profile could almost perfectly be realized by the combination of different preparations of gentamicin and clindamycin palmitate loaded on porous hydroxyapatite (Endobon®, Fig. **3**). The composition shown in Table **2** resulted in a release of gentamicin and clindamycin for serum and buffer as shown in Figures **4** and **5**, respectively.

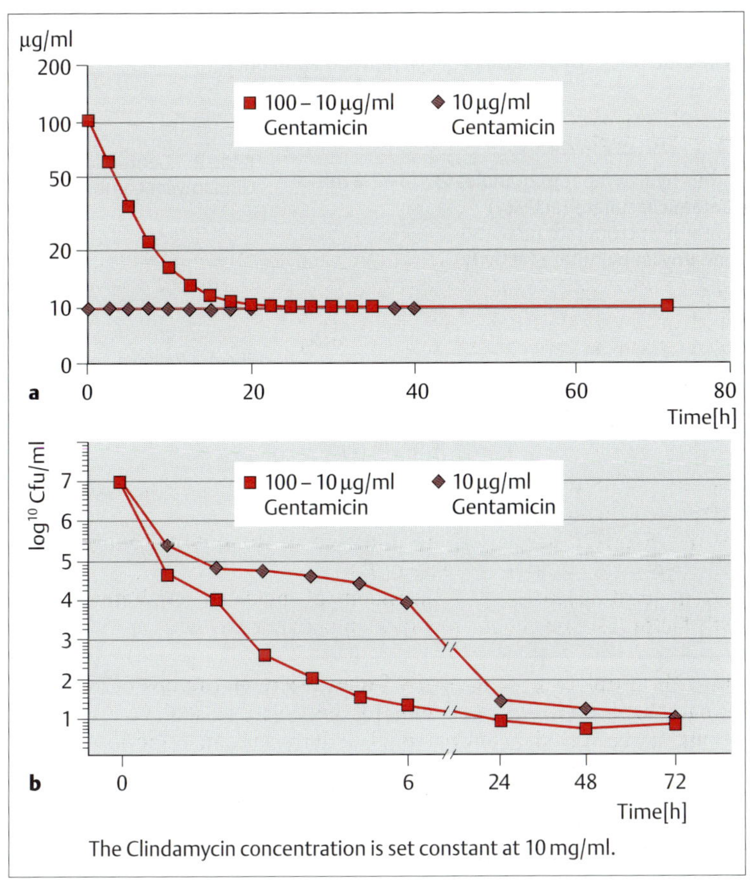

Fig. **2**
(**a**) Concentration curves of gentamicin and clindamycin.
(**b**) Bactericidal activity against *Staphylococcus aureus* at 2 different kinetics of gentamicin in combination with clindamycin.

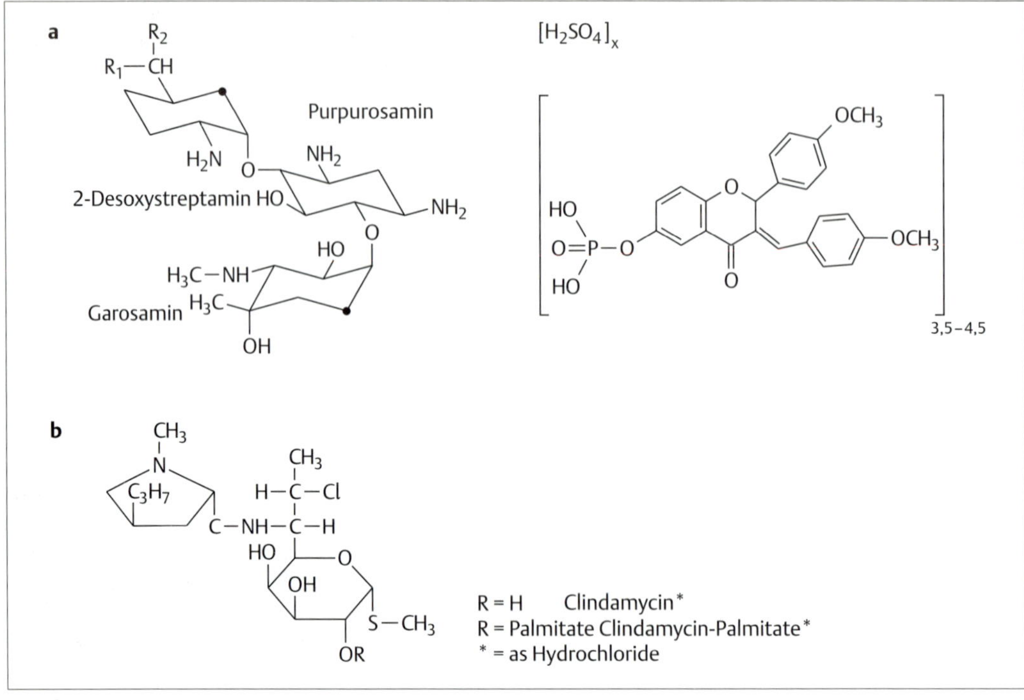

Fig. 3   (a) Structures of gentamicin antibiotics. (b) Structures of clindamycin antibiotics.

Bone substitute:	1.0 g	porous hydroxyapatite granules ∅ 1.4–2.8 mm
Antibiotics:	4.0 mg	Gentamicin sulfate (activity)
	14.0 mg	Gentamicin crobefate (activity)
	20.0 mg	Clindamycin palmitate (activity)

Table 2   Gentamicin-clindamycin combinations

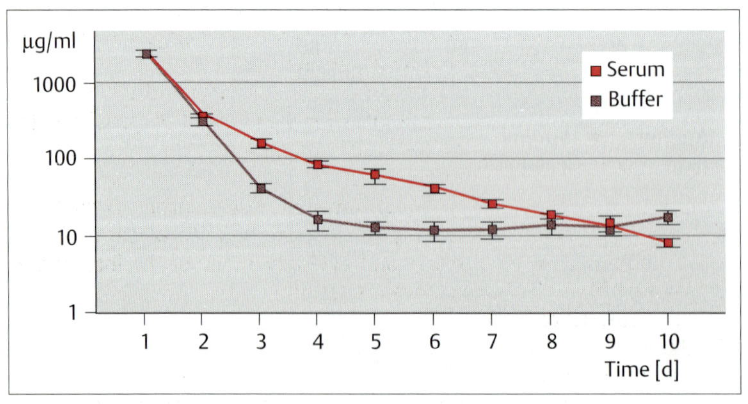

Fig. 4   Release of gentamicin in serum and buffer.

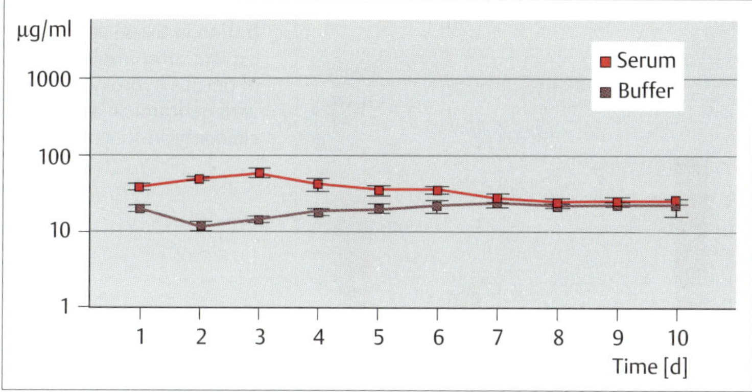

Fig. **5** Release of clindamycin in serum and buffer.

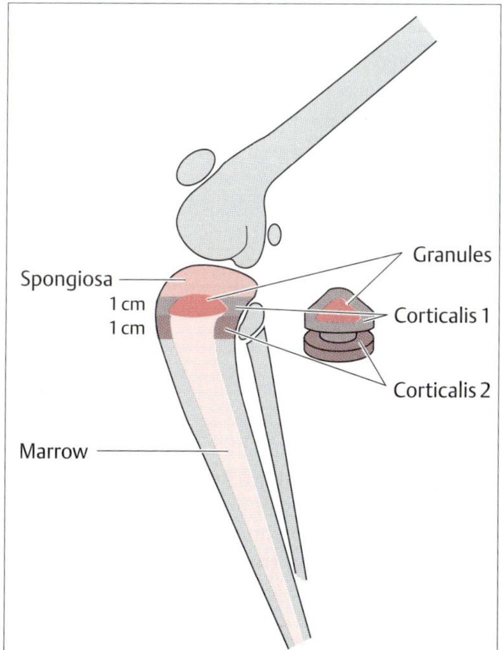

Fig. **6** Implantation in proximal tibia of rabbits.

After implantation of 1 g of antibiotic-loaded porous hydroxyapatite into the proximal tibia of rabbits (schematic drawing in Fig. **6**) only trace amounts of gentamicin could be detected in the serum and no clindamycin could be detected at all. This result again demonstrates that local application of antibiotic carriers typically leads to a neglectable systemic drug burden with the accompanied low risk of toxicity. On the other hand, the local antibiotic concentrations in the tissues surrounding the implantation site reach rather high levels, which are maintained after 7 and 14 days, respectively (Fig. **7**). Within the 7 days interval most of the gentamicin has already been released whereas approximately 50% of the applied clindamycin is retained even after 2 weeks.

In spite of the high local drug concentrations at the implantation site the histological evaluation of the 2-week explants revealed a beginning bony integration of the bone substitute material. It can be concluded, therefore, that both the applied antibiotics are very well tolerated locally and that bone regeneration is not significantly impaired.

Conclusion

For the development of bone substitute materials as antibiotic carriers the available knowledge and technology allows us

- to select appropriate drugs or drug combinations that cover the relevant bacterial spectra of selected indications almost completely, and
- to design antibiotic release profiles which optimally exploit the activity of the selected drugs and take advantage of the local mode of administration.

Perspectives

At present, bone substitute materials are used in less than 10% of surgical procedures requiring defect filling. This figure will increase significantly.

As the indications for bone substitute materials differ greatly, the request for improved prop-

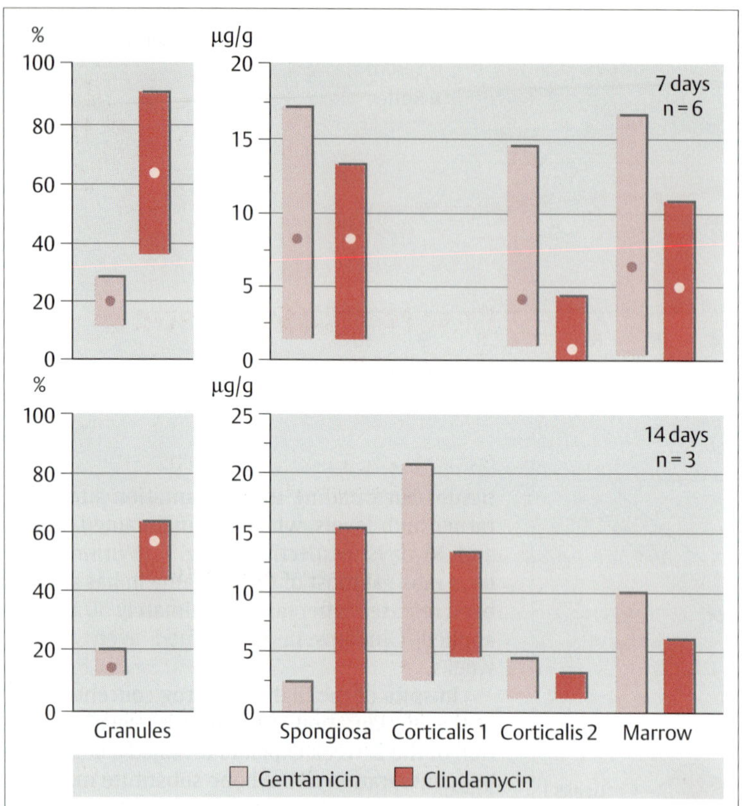

Fig. 7   Antibiotic concentration in tissue and explant after implantation of porous hydroxyapatite with gentamicin and clindamycin.

erties will be intensified in order to meet the special requirements within certain indications.

Today, the technology is available to develop fixed combinations of bone substitutes with potent antimicrobial agents that could enable surgeons to treat bone infections much more efficiently.

For the development of fixed combinations of bone substitutes with osteoinductive proteins several scientific questions still have to be answered and some technological problems have to be solved. Among the alternative approaches to stimulate bone regeneration the combination of bone substitutes with appropriate drugs on the spot will be an attractive way out, as soon as such drugs are available.

4

Resorbable Synthetic Polymers

Bioresorbable Synthetic Polymers and their Operation Field

M. Vert

Introduction

It is within the last two decades that people have tried to take advantage of the degradation of polymers for therapeutic purposes. As a matter of fact, the parenteral compartments of a mammalian organism are practically close to the entrance or the exit of high molecular weight materials because of the barriers constituted by endothelial cells, mucosa, and skin. Therefore, it is critical that polymeric prosthetic devices be bioresorbable if they are to be used temporarily to help the normal processes by which a living organism effects self-repair. A variety of synthetic polymers have been reported to degrade under conditions modelling body fluids and mammalian tissues. However, the degradation of polymeric materials is always a complex phenomenon which depends on many factors, especially *in vivo* (Vert, 1990). Until now, no consensual terminology has been accepted world-wide to distinguish the different ways by which a polymeric material can degrade, namely purely physical degradation, as is the case when the macromolecules go into solution, or chemical degradation, the latter involving repeated cleavages of the macromolecule. In order to distinguish the different levels of degradation, we have proposed to use the term *"degradable"* to define a polymeric material which falls into pieces because of macromolecule cleavages, i.e., via chemical routes. Accordingly, *"biodegradation"* is now regarded as reflecting the fact that macromolecule degradation is mediated by living systems such as enzymes, cells, tissues, or organs. However, biodegradation reflects a mechanism of chain attack but does not say anything about the fate of degradation by-products. In order to characterize those polymers which totally resorb by excretion or by assimilation to form biomass via enzymatic processes, we recommended the use of the word *"bioresorbable"*. Accordingly, this word normally applies to polymeric materials whose degradation by-products have been shown to be totally eliminated from a living organism through natural pathways, i.e., either by kidney filtration or because of metabolization (Vert et al., 1984).

Many polymers can degrade or biodegrade in a mammalian body. However, only a small number of these polymers can fulfil the requirements related to a given temporary therapeutic application and those related to bioresorption. On the other hand, the number of potential applications is rather large. For example, one can mention suturing, internal bone fracture fixation, reconstructive substitutes, sheets for preventing adhesion, and even blood vessel prostheses. Another attractive type of application of these polymers deals with the concept of controlled drug delivery via parenteral routes. Various systems are currently being investigated, namely implants, micro- and nanoparticles, aggregates, micelles, and even macromolecular prodrugs and polymeric drugs (Vert, 1986). It is worth noting that bioresorbable polymers can be of interest in orthopedic surgery either to make temporary prosthetic devices (plates, screws, nails, pins, etc.), to make drug delivery systems, or to make both as in the case of medicated temporary prosthetic devices. The possibility of medication by combination with drugs followed by slow release is one of the main advantages of polymeric biomaterials. The control of the release can be achieved by diffusion, by degradation, and by both. Of course, many polymeric compounds of natural origin (proteins, polysaccharides) have been or are used as degradable, biodegradable, or bioresorbable biomaterials. However, they exhibit various major shortcomings. They are difficult to process thermally. They have a limited range of properties. They raise a high risk of immune response because of their animal and sometimes human origins. Last but not least, they now raise a risk of infection related to the development of viral diseases.

Poly(glycolic acid)
PGA
$$-[O-CH_2-CO]_n-$$

Poly(L-lactic acid)
PLA100
$$-[O-\underset{\underset{CH_3}{|}}{\overset{\overset{H}{|}}{C}}-CO]_n-$$

Poly(lactic acid) stereocopolymers
PLAx
$$-[O-\underset{\underset{CH_3}{|}}{\overset{\overset{H}{|}}{C}}-CO]_m-[O-\underset{\underset{H}{|}}{\overset{\overset{CH_3}{|}}{C}}-CO]_p-$$

Poly(L-lactic acid-co-glycolic acid)
PLAxGA100-x
$$-[O-\underset{\underset{CH_3}{|}}{\overset{\overset{H}{|}}{C}}-CO]_m-[O-CH_2-CO]_p-$$

Poly(L-lactic-co-D-lactic-co-glycolic acids) terpolymers
PLAxGAy
$$-[O-\underset{\underset{CH_3}{|}}{\overset{\overset{H}{|}}{C}}-CO]_m-[O-\underset{\underset{H}{|}}{\overset{\overset{CH_3}{|}}{C}}-CO]_p-[O-CH_2-CO]_q-$$

Fig. 1 Chemical structures of glycolic and lactic acid polymers.

Among the few synthetic polymers which have been recognized as bioresorbable so far, aliphatic polyesters of the poly(α-hydroxy acid)-type which derive from metabolites like lactic acid enantiomers (L-LA and D-LA) and glycolic acid (GA) (Fig. 1), are receiving increasing attention because of their remarkable biocompatibility and versatility (Vert, 1989). The versatility of PLA/GA polymers is primarily due to the poly(α-hydroxy acid) backbone which allows property adjustments either by combination of lactic and glycolic repeating units via copolymerization or by combination of L- and D-isomers of chiral lactic acid (L-LA and D-LA, respectively) by stereocopolymerization or both.

Basically, only highly stereoregular L-lactic-rich poly(lactic acids), which degrade very slowly, are able to fulfil lifetime requirements of fracture healing and are thus usable for fracture fixation (Vert, 1984). In contrast, members of the family leading to intrinsically amorphous compounds degrade more rapidly and are preferable for controlled drug delivery.

The degradation behavior of aliphatic polyesters, in particular of LA/GA polymers, has been investigated extensively. Factors such as molecular weight (MW), MW distribution, and polymer morphology have been identified as playing important roles insofar as polymer degradation is concerned (Vert, 1990). Actually, they play critical roles for polymer properties and drug delivery phenomena as well. Semicrystalline stereoregular poly(lactic acids) have been known for a long time to degrade faster in amorphous regions than in crystalline ones, the degradation being autocatalyzed due to the increase of the amount of catalytic carboxylic acid end groups present in the polymeric mass when macromolecules degrade. This mechanism was said to be qualitatively the same for all the aliphatic polyesters despite a range of structures and morphologies. However, many details remain confusing and sometimes controversial when one tries to analyse the literature data. Hydrolytic degradation was reported in the past as occurring in the bulk by most authors and through surface erosion by some others. Most of the remarks present in literature are of interest. The main problem is twofold: first, polymer degradation depends very much on the grade of the polymer itself, second, investigators did not pay enough attention to the complexity of the polymer structures which condition this grade. In many instances, properties of polymers are discussed on the basis of compounds whose structures are unknown, or simply not reported. This problem was first underlined in 1981 (Vert et al., 1981) and still exists today. The situation is even worse now because of the possibility for anyone to buy commercially available PLA/GA polymers of different grades and of different ages, sometimes with rather limited information about the initial properties. Nevertheless, it is now generally admitted that the initial chain cleavage of LA/GA polymers is hydrolytic and not enzymatic.

PLAGA Synthesis

PLAGA polymers of biomedical interest are presently synthesized by ring opening polymerization of cyclic dimers, namely lactides and glycolide. It is because of the chirality of the lactide ring which contains two asymmetric carbon atoms that one can diversify very much the properties via stereocopolymerization and copolymerization (Fig. 1). The lactide and glycolide polymerization can be initiated by many compounds. Only three are presently used industrially: Zn metal and Zn lactate (Phusilines from Phusis, France) and stannous octoate by all the other companies offering marketed PLAGA polymers. The number of companies which sell devices commercially for bone surgery is very small, these devices being either machined from blocks or injection moulded. These two processing methods usually do not lead to similar morphologies when one deals with the semicrystalline members of the PLAGA family.

General Degradation Mechanism

Two decades ago, the hydrolytic degradation of aliphatic polyesters of the PLAGA-type was regarded as depending primarily on the kinetics of the chemical cleavage of an ester according to the well known reaction:

$$R\text{-}COO\text{-}R' + H_2O \rightarrow RCOOH + R'OH$$

A major improvement was the discovery of the effect of autocatalysis by the acid terminal chain fragments which leads to a dramatic increase in the rate of degradation as degradation advances (Pitt et al., 1981). It was also recognized early that degradation is much faster in amorphous domains than in crystalline ones, mostly because water penetration is easier within a disordered network of polymer chains. For the same reason plus the consequences of the mobility of chain segments, degradation is faster in amorphous domains above the glass transition point than below. However, it is with the consideration of the degradation mechanism of large devices (Li, 1995) that the principles of the degradation of aliphatic polyesters became clear and allowed us to account for the unexpected findings listed in Table 1.

From a general viewpoint, the degradation mechanism of PLAGA polymers depends totally on diffusion-reaction phenomena. First, degradation causes an increase in the number of carboxylic chain ends which are known to autocatalyze the ester hydrolysis. Second, only oligomers which are soluble in the surrounding aqueous medium can escape from the matrix. As the aging time increases, soluble oligomers which are close to the surface can leach out before total degradation whereas those which are located well inside the matrix remain entrapped so that all of them contribute to the autocatalytic degradation. The resulting slower surface degradation yields a skin composed of less degraded polymer surrounding a core whose fate and aspect depend very much on chain gross composition and on unit distribution. It also very well explains why large devices degrade faster than small ones (Grizzi et al., 1995).

Degradation-induced crystallization in quenched crystallizable PLAGA below Tg

Degradation-induced crystallization of non-crystallizable PLAGA

Unusual size-dependence (large devices degrading faster than small ones)

Occasional catalysis by acidic additives or loads

Occasional catalysis by basic additives or loads

Occasional appearance of bimodal SEC traces with degradation

Occasional appearance of dramatically degradation-resistant crystalline residues

Occasional formation of hollow structures

Initiator-dependence of the properties of polymers obtained by ring opening polymerization of cyclic dimers

Slower degradation of porous devices as compared with plain ones

Table **1** Unexpected findings observed during the degradation of PLA/GA aliphatic polyesters in aqueous media or *in vivo*

From the diffusion-reaction mechanism mentioned above, one can identify a few basic parameters which govern the whole hydrolytic degradation process of PLAGA polymers, namely:

- The *hydrolysis rate constant* of the α-alkanoate ester bond: we have recently found that this rate constant does not depend on the configurational structure when polymers are in solution in dioxane. In contrast, hydrolysis has been shown to depend very much on unit distribution and sequencing via the consequences of these structural parameters on the morphology of the compounds in the solid state,
- The *diffusion coefficient of water* within the array of poly(α-alkanoate) molecules: an ester bond engaged within a crystalline array is much more resistant than the same bond engaged within an amorphous domain.
- The *diffusion coefficient of chain fragments* within the polymeric matrix: the smaller the fragments the greater is the diffusion coefficient. However, even the diffusion of the smaller fragments is a slow process.
- The *solubility of degradation products,* generally oligomers, within the surrounding liquid medium from which penetrating water is issued.

Any additional factors such as temperature, additives in the polymeric matrix, additives in the surrounding medium, pH, buffering capacity, size and processing history, quenching or annealing, steric hindrance, porosity, etc. (Vert, 1990), affect the general balance through their effects on the main factors listed above.

From the viewpoint of surgical applications, the structure- and size-dependent release of soluble compounds as well as the formation of particles occurring sooner or later during the degradation process well accounts for the secondary inflammatory response of variable intensity which had been regarded for long as a mystery by surgeons (Vert et al., 1992).

Recent Findings Concerning the Effects of the Polymerization Initiator

At present, there are two main initiator systems which are used industrially. One, stannous octoate is used world-wide because it leads to fast polymerization, high yields, high molar masses, and has been approved by FDA in USA. The other, zinc metal, is used in France to make internal bone and ligament fixation devices because it leads to good compromises with respect to biocompatibility, biofunctionality specifications, and injection moulding requirements. Although this was never explicitly stated, literature data suggested the existence of differences in structural, degradation, and biological behaviors between the resulting two types of PLA polymers.

We have recently shown that the two initiators, which are both configuration-respecting, lead to stereocopolymers with different chiral repeating unit distributions, depending on polymerization conditions and transesterification reactions (Schwach et al., 1994). For the sake of securing a significant comparative approach in spite of the differences in configurational structures, selection was made of two polymers with rather close molar masses, polydispersity indexes, and transesterification coefficients, although it was impossible to compare strictly identical compounds. Both PLA50 polymers were synthesised starting from the same lactide monomer. They were both processed to $10 \times 10 \times 2$ mm parallel-sided specimens by compression moulding. This size and shape is known to give rise to heterogeneous degradation. Insofar as water absorption is concerned, the Zn-initiated polymer appears much more hydrophilic than the Sn-initiated one. Both compounds led to heterogeneous degradation. The Zn-initiated PLA50 was slightly ahead of the Sn-initiated one, the dramatic weight loss characteristics of heterogeneous degradation occurring at 900 and 1,200 hours post immersion, respectively (Schwach, 1996).

Differences were correlated to rather distinct mechanisms of polymerization. Sn-octoate initiation was shown to lead to more hydrophobic matrices because most macromolecules bear alcohol chain ends esterified by octanoic acid residues whereas Zn-metal yielded OH-free chain ends (Schwach et al., 1996).

Furthermore, it was shown that stannous octoate yielded hydrophobic initiator residues (stannous hydroxyoctoate and/or stannous hydroxylactate) which remained entrapped within the Sn-initiated polymer matrix because of the poor solubility in the aging medium. All these particular features merged to make Sn-initiated matrices more hydrophobic and thus more resistant to degradation (Vert et al., 1992).

Conclusions

The initial morphological characteristics of bioresorbable plastic devices derived from PLA/GA members with stereo-ordered polymer chains are of great practical interest for biomedical applications. However, one has to keep in mind that both retention of mechanical property and bioresorption depend very much on the origin of the polymers. Our recent advances in the understanding of the degradation of LA/GA polymers, namely the discovery of the surface/center differentiation and that of degradation-induced morphology and composition changes, brought about new insights which are of great interest to predict, at least qualitatively, the fate of implanted polymers. However, the main message of this contribution will be that the biofunctionality, the bioresorption, and the inflammatory responses depend on many factors, especially the polymer chain configurational substructure, the synthesis route, the processing method, and the thermal history. If one wants to really compare polymers bearing the same name but having different origins, information has to be supplied on the chemical composition of the polymer chains or of the parent monomer feed, the molecular weight, and the molecular weight polydispersity as they are deduced from SEC chromatograms. Actually, these characteristics are no longer sufficient and factors like size, stereosequence distribution, morphology, thermal and storage histories, etc., have to be mentioned too. This is not being done in the literature, thus explaining the discrepancies one can find so often between the reported clinical behaviors of bioresorbable polymeric devices.

Acknowledgements

The author is indebted to all his co-workers who contributed to collect the knowledge reported herein.

References

Grizzi I, Garreau H, Li S, Vert M. Biomaterials 1995; 16: 305.

Li SM, Vert M. In: Scott G, Gilead D (eds.). Degradable Polymers: Principles and Applications. Chapman & Hall, London 1995: 43.

Pitt CG, Gratzel MM, Kimmel GL, Surles J, Schindler A. Biomaterials 1981; 2: 215.

Schwach G. PhD thesis, University Montpellier 1, France, February 1996.

Schwach G, Coudane J, Engel R, Vert M. Polym. Bull. 1994; 32: 617.

Schwach G, Coudane J, Engel R, Vert M. Polym. Bull. 1996; 37: 771.

Vert M. Polyvalent polymeric drug carriers. In: Buck S (ed.). CRC Critical Review – Therapeutic Drug Carrier systems. CRC Press, Boca Raton 1986; 2: 291.

Vert M. Angew. Makromol. Chem. 1989; 166/167: 155.

Vert M, Chabot F, Leray J, Christel P. Bioresorbable polymers for bone surgery. Makromol. Chem. 1981; (Supp. 5): 30.

Vert M. In: Barenberg SA, Brash JL, Narayan R, Redpath AE (eds.). Biodegradable Materials. CRC Press, Boca Raton, FL 1990: p. 11.

Vert M, Christel P, Chabot F, Leray J. In: Hastings GW, Ducheyne P. (eds.). Macromolecular Materials. CRC Press, Boca Raton 1984; Chap. 4: 119.

Vert M, Li Suming, Spenlehauer G, Guérin Ph. J. Mater Sci.: Mater. Med. 1992; 3: 432.

Bioresorbable Polymers as Materials in Osteosynthesis

P. Patka, T. E. Otto, M. van der Elst, H. J. Th. M. Haarman, F. C. Bakker

Introduction

Most of the implants used for the stabilization of fractures in current operative fracture treatment are made from stainless steel or more recently from titanium. These metal implants became widely used in fracture surgery because of their easy handling, easy production and availability, and relatively low prices.

However, metal implants are also associated with many problems. The stress-shielding phenomenon or stress-protection related atrophy of bone, the risk of infection and allergic or even toxic reactions are well recognized complications in operative fracture treatment using metal implants (Schuster, 1972).

Because of these hazards, related to the use of non-degradable metal implants, there is a necessity of an additional surgery to remove the implant after fracture healing.

The use of a bioresorbable fracture fixation device will make this additional surgical procedure, surgery for removal of the implant, unnecessary. This shall save the patient from considerable psychological and physical discomfort. And last but not least there will also be an economic benefit from omitting an additional surgical procedure and concomitant disability.

All surgeons are, more or less, familiar with resorbable sutures. Plain silk or metal sutures, which are of course non-degradable, already deserved their place in history. Since the use of resorbable sutures, started in 1970 and becoming common in surgical practice in the 80's, many different types of resorbable surgical materials and implants have been developed. This innovation in the field of materials used for fixation of fractures, was a result of emerging technology, especially in biomechanics and materials science (Patka et al., 1995).

These developments resulted not only in new designs of mechanical devices but also in new materials like biodegradable and bioresorbable polymers. It is not surprising that the first bioresorbable fracture fixation materials were derived from resorbable sutures.

Bioresorbable materials, polymeric or composite materials retain their supporting properties after their implantation in living tissue from days to months. These materials degrade gradually into a tissue compatible component which will be absorbed and finally exported out of the body. An example of such a degradation and resorption is a polyglycolide which is a polymer of glycolic acid. This polymer will be depolymerized in the human body. The final stage of degradation is resorption and elimination which occurs when glycolide is converted into carbon dioxide and pyruvate which enters into the tricarboxylic acid cycle (Krebs cycle) via the acetylation of coenzyme A. During this final stage the major elimination of PGA occurs through respiration (carbon dioxide) with only minor elimination via urine and/or feces. This procedure starts within a few hours after implantation and will be finished, depending on the amount of the material implanted, within a few days up to 3 months. By combining two or more different polymers, like in PLLA/PGA copolymer, it is possible to speed up or to delay the biodegradation time. Also the molecular weight has an influence on the degradation time. A higher molecular weight of a polymer implant will result in a longer degradation time and a low molecular weight will result in fast degradation of an implant.

Since the introduction of synthetic polymers several decades ago, a variety of materials with differing degradation time, mechanical properties, and shape has been developed (Hollinger and Schmitz, 1987; Patka et al., 1995; Tormala et al., 1991).

Thus, today biodegradable implants from different origins are used as suture materials, implants for fracture fixation, drug delivery systems, vascular prostheses, and in other applications.

Biodegradable polymer used as an implant for fracture stabilization was first described by Kulkani et al. (1971). Since then, biodegradable implants have demonstrated good biocompatibility with bone tissue in animal studies and since 1984 also in clinical trials on operative fracture treatment (Christel et al., 1984; Dijkema et al., 1993; Matsuse et al., 1991; Otto et al., 1995; Perren, 1979). From these reports it seems that the mechanical properties of the polymers show a considerable variation. The distribution of molecular weights plays an important role. The crystallinity, the amount of free monomers, and the stereotactic configuration are other factors that influence the mechanical properties of the biodegradable material (Bergsma et al., 1996; Elst et al., 1996).

A biodegradable material used for fracture fixation must supply the injured bone with sufficient support for a sufficient length of time. In several animal studies, polylactic acid (PLLA) pins or screws have been used as fracture fixation devices. The ultimate strength of PLLA rods resembles the ultimate strength of cortical bone, i.e., 10–150 MPa. Polylactic acid with a high mean molecular weight (260,000), a low degree of crystallinity, and a small amount of free monomers may contribute to a development of a biodegradable intramedullary nail for fracture fixation (Daniels et al., 1990; Elst et al., 1995; Elst, 1997).

Biocompatibility

The development and application of implants in fracture surgery made it necessary to give increasing attention to the materials used for the manufacturing of such implants. These materials, which are also referred to as biomaterials, have to meet certain chemical, physical, and biological requirements in order to ensure optimum and lasting function of the implant and success of the implantation procedure. The chemical and physical requirements include such properties as strength, wearing friction behavior, and corrosion resistance, as well as workability and sterilizability. Acceptance by living tissue and stability within the body constitute important biological requirements. Biocompatibility is determined by the extent of chemical and biological interaction between host and implant, and the stability (mechanical integrity) of the implant.

A compatible implant would have no effect on the adjacent tissue, the nearby cells would show no abnormalities, no variant cell types would appear, there would be no inflammatory reactions, and there would be no cell necrosis. The histology of the tissue surrounding the implant would be altogether normal (Otto et al., 1994). The implant recognized by the recipient as a foreign body will be isolated by encapsulation. Commonly, the thickness of the encapsulating fibrous tissue membrane is often taken as a measure of the compatibility of the implant in relation to the surrounding tissue. The thinner the membrane, the better is the compatibility of the implant.

Current Biodegradable and Bioresorbable Polymers

Most bioresorbable fracture fixation materials are derived from the resorbable suture materials. At present, the most important degradable implant materials are:
- Poly-L-lactic acid (PLLA),
- Poly-DL-lactic acid (PDLLA),
- Polyglycolic acid (PGA),
- Polydioxanone (PDS),
- Polyorthoester (POE), and
- Poly-C-capralactone (PCL).

The screws and pins made from SR-PLLA were used in operative fracture treatment in different sites of human body. The ankle fracture, olecranon fracture, distal radial fracture, and patellar fracture are the most common sites for the use of biodegradable implants. In these fractures the amount of cortical bone is not a problem for torsional strength of the SR-PLLA screw. When the operative technique is applied in a proper way there will be only rare breaks of the screwhead occurring during its insertion in the fracture site.

But there are other problems and these problems are related to tissue reaction and biocompatibility. The so-called sterile sinus, which is a swelling observed at the implantation site in the first few weeks, was seen almost only in polyglycolide implants. On the other hand, implants made from PLA showed, in areas covered by thin subcutaneous tissue, an increasing swelling from 3 up to 5 years after implantation. The problem is caused by a crystalline remnant of degraded PLLA material surrounded by dense fibrous tissue and was reported by Bos in 1993. The intra- and extracellular degradation rate of these crystalline particles is very slow, as these particles were found in tissues 5 years after implantation (Bergsma et al., 1996).

The clinical significance of this phenomenon is not clear yet. In places with a sufficient soft tissue cover, no problems are reported. In intraosseal placed PLA implants, like in case of ankle fractures, no significant problems were notified. However, in cases where plates or another extraosseal implantation is necessary one should be aware of this late reaction and the associated problems (Eitenmuller et al., 1987).

Bioresorbable bone fixation implants are in clinical use during the last 12 years. First implants were used in operative treatment of ankle fractures (Rokkanen et al., 1985). Fractures located in or around the joint are a good indication for the use of bioresorbable implants (Fig. **1**).

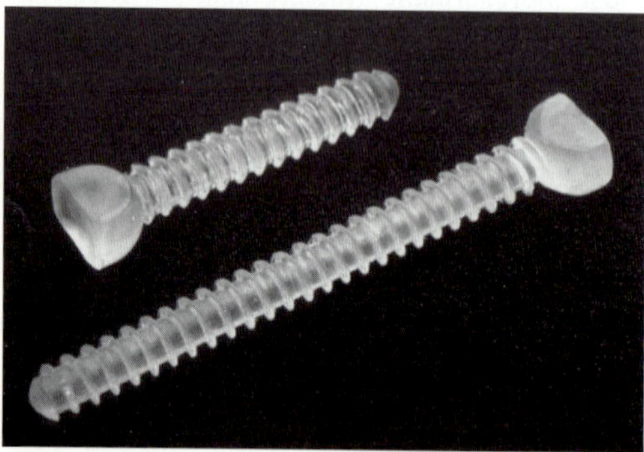

Fig. **1**   The Biofix® screw which can be used for stabilization of a fracture.

Until now, the most important limitation for use is that the presently available resorbable implants cannot be used for the treatment of fractures of long cortical bones. Also a limited variability of implant designs is a restriction for more extended clinical use as well as the late tissue reaction produced by crystalline remnants of some degraded polymers.

And last but not least, economical reasons are still an important factor for the limited use of degradable materials in surgery. Because of the ongoing development, additional costs with manufacturing, storage and sterilization and the costs of education of surgeons in handling a new material, the biodegradable implant is initially far more expensive than the implant made from metal.

However, the basic natural resources like aliphatic polyesters or alpha-hydroxy acid derivates like polylactic acid and polyglycolic acid for bio-

resorbable implants are cheap and available in unlimited quantity. This together with improvement in bioengineering and increasing consumption of these devices will result in a lower implant price in the near future.

Some precautions and restrictions for application of biodegradable implants, especially concerning the resorbability of high crystalline remnants of PLLA, must be included for some indications like fractures covered by only thin subcutaneous tissue. More research and especially long-term experience would be desirable especially on this subject.

Up till now, there are no major problems referring to the use of biodegradable implants of a limited amount of material in operative fracture treatment. The advantage is that there is no necessity for additional surgery to remove these implants and that osteoporosis and other mechanical problems associated with application of a rigid metal implant can be avoided.

Resorbable polymer implants are promising options for fixation of fractured bones in trauma surgery. However, some problems remain to be solved prior to general use of these implants in surgery. Examples of these problems are:
1. The progress of the resorption process,
2. The control of mechanical properties,
3. The effect of the decreased pH,
4. The burst phenomenon, and
5. The possibility of mutagenicity.

It is obvious that the optimal degradation characteristics of an implant for tissue protection and for improving the tissue strength during the healing process of bone fractures still have to be found.

Currently, limited use of presently available degradable implants is allowed to those who are able and willing to change their routine treatment of fractures. They have to treat fractures within the limitations of the presently available degradable implants.

References

Bergsma JE, Bos RRM, Rozema FR, Jong W de, Boering G. Biocompatibility of intraosseously implanted predegraded poly(lactide): an animal study. J Mater Sci Mater Med 1996; 7: 1 – 7.

Christel PS, Vert M, Chabot F et al. Polylactic acid for intra-medullary plugging. Biomaterials and Biomechanics 1983. Elseviers Science Publishers, 1984.

Daniels AU, Chang MKO, Andriano KP. Mechanical properties of biodegradable polymers and composites proposed for internal fixation of bone. J Applied Biomat 1990; 1 : 57 – 8.

Dijkema ARA, Elst M van der, Breederveld RS, Verspui G, Patka P, Haarman HJThM. The surgical treatment of fracture dislocations of the ankle joint with biodegradable implants. J Trauma 1993; 34: 82 – 5.

Eitenmuller J, Gerlach KL, Schmickal T, Muhr G. Semirigide Plattenosteosynthesen unter Verwendung absorbierbaren Polymere als temporäre Implantate. Chirurg 1987; 58: 831 – 9.

Elst M van der, Dijkema ARA, Klein CPAT, Patka P, Haarman HJThM. Tissue reaction on PLLA versus stainless steel interlocking nails for fracture fixation. An animal study. Biomaterials 1995; 16: 103 – 6.

Elst M van der, Kuiper I, Klein CPAT, Patka P, Haarman HJThM. The burst phenomenon, an animal model simulating the long-term tissue response on PLLA interlocking nails. J Biomed Mater Res 1996; 30: 139 – 43.

Elst M van der. Biodegradable interlocking nail. PhD thesis, Vrije Universiteit Amsterdam, 1997.

Hollinger JO, Schmitz JP. Restoration of bone discontinuities in dogs using a biodegradable implant. J Oral and Maxillofacial Surg 1987; 45: 594 – 600.

Kulkarni RK, Moore EG, Hegyeli AF, Leonard F. Biodegradable poly(lactic acid) polymers. J Biomed Mater Res 1971; 5: 169 – 81.

Matsusue Y, Yamamuro T, Yoshii S, Oka M, et al. Biodegradable screw fixation of rabbit tibia proximal osteotomies. J Applied Biomat 1991; 2: 1 – 12.

Otto TE, Patka P, Haarman HJThM. Formation of a bony sheath around intramedullary implanted polylactic acid wire. Osteo Int 1995; 2: 129 – 33.

Otto TE, Patka P, Haarman HJThM, Klein CPAT, Vriesde R. Intramedullary bone formation after polylactic acid wire implantation. J Mater Sci Mater Med 1994; 5: 407 – 11.

Patka P, Haarman HJThM, Elst M van der. Bone substitution and bone repair in trauma surgery. In: Wise DL (ed.). Encyclopedic Handbook of Biomaterials and Bioengineering. Part B Applications. Marcel Dekker Inc., New York 1995: 639 – 64.

Perren SM. Physical and biological aspects of fracture healing with special reference to internal fixation. Clinical Orthop and Rel Res 1979; 138.

Rokkanen P, Bostman O, Vainionpaa S, et al. Biodegradable implants in fracture fixation: early results of treatment of fractures of the ankle. The Lancet 1985: 1422 – 4.

Schuster J. Die Metallose. Chirurg 1972; 43: 114 – 6.

Tormala P, Vasenius J, Vainiopaa S, et al. Ultra-high-strength absorbable self-reinforced polyglycolide (SR-PGA) composite rods for internal fixation of bone fractures. J Biomed Mater Res 1991; 25: 1 – 21.

Properties of the Biomaterial "Polyactive".
In vivo Animal Studies and the First Clinical Results

S. K. Bulstra, R. Kuijer, S. J. M. Bouwmeester, D. J. Bakker, C. A. van Blitterswijk,
N. H. M. Hoefnagels, R. Van den Munckhof

Introduction

Recently, a new material was discovered that proved to be biocompatible, bioerodible, and osteoconductive (Bucholz et al., 1987; Geesink, 1992; Huiskes et al., 1984; Muschler et al., 1993). This material, trademarked as Polyactive, is a polyetherpolyester segmented block copolymer, composed of a soft segment, polyethylene oxide (PEO), and a hard segment, polybutylene terephthalate (PBT).

Based on the same compounds, a whole range of copolymers with different degradation characteristics can be obtained by varying the PEO/PBT ratio. The PEO component stands for the bone-bonding properties of the material, provided it is used in relatively high amounts; 60% PEO or higher. Also with increasing amounts of PEO the degradation speed is increased (Bakker et al., 1990; Blitterswijk, 1992; Blitterswijk et al., 1991).

Bone formation is preceded by selective absorption of calcium in the hydrogel polyactive. PA has a spongy appearance and it is easy to manipulate (Blitterswijk et al., 1993, Blitterswijk et al., 1991, Blitterswijk et al., 1992).

In this study some of the extensive research that was performed with Polyactive in rabbit experiments will be described. The research performed resulted in some clinical applications of which the first results will be presented.

Experiments with Polyactive in the Rabbit

In this study Polyactive cylinders (70/30 as well as 60/40) were used to fill defects in the proximal femur and in the trochlea of the knee, where defects into the subchondral bone were made. The goal of this study was to quantify the osteoconductive properties of Polyactive in different bone locations such as the cortex, the medullary canal, and the trabecular subchondral bone.

Materials and Methods

Polyactive (PA 70/30 and 60/40) cylinders were manufactured and supplied by HC Implants bv., Leiden, The Netherlands. The average pore diameter was 300 ± 150 pm; the diameter of the interconnecting pores was 100 ± 50 pm. These diameters have been shown to be optimal for the ingrowing of bone. The cylinders were 4 mm in diameter and had a length of 5 mm. All PA cylinders were sterilized by gamma irradiation (25 KGy) at Gammamaster, Ede, The Netherlands.

Sixty-four female New Zealand White Rabbits of about six months old were used, weighing between 3.5 and 4.5 kg. the rabbits were anesthetized using ketamine hydrochloride (100 mg/kg) and diazepam (8 mg/kg). The left knee was opened through a medial parapatellar incision and the patella was dislocated laterally. A bore hole of 4 mm in diameter was made in the facies patellaris of the femur. A PA cylinder was placed in the bore hole. In the right knee a sham operation was performed without drilling the bore hole.

The right femur was exposed laterally by pushing off the musculature ventrally. the periosteum was put aside and approximately 1.5 cm below the major trochanter a bore hole of 4 mm diameter was made. The PA cylinder was placed here. Again, the contralateral side was used as a control; a bore hole was made without placing a PA 70/30 cylinder. The cylinders were placed in the defect of the femur up to the contralateral cortex. Four groups of sixteen rabbits were sacrificed after respectively four, eight, twenty-six, and fifty-two weeks. The animals were killed using an overdose of thiopental intravenously. Both knees and femurs were dissected and fixed in 4% phosphate-buffered formaldehyde. The specimens were dehydrated through a series of acetone/alcohol solutions and embedded in methyl methacrylate. Sections of 10 µm were cut using an innerlock diamond saw and stained with methylene blue and basic fuchsin. To determine the percentage of area occupied by implant material, exudate cells, fibrous tissue, and bone, we used an image analyser (Quantimet 570 C, Leica Cambridge Ltd, Cambridge, UK). For statistical analysis data were compared using the one way ANOVA test.

Results

From the sixty-four rabbits that were operated, nine died or had to be killed before the end of the experiment. Causes of death were either pneumonia in three cases, meningitis in one case, or fractures at the level of the bore hole in five cases. One rabbit developed an osteomyelitis and was withdrawn from this study.

Already four weeks after implantation some bone formation was seen in the PA cylinders placed in the trochlea. After 8 weeks about 28% of the pores were filled with bone trabeculi and after 52 weeks this percentage was reduced to 14.5%, which proved to be comparable to the amount of bone found in normal subchondral bone. In the cortex of the femur, after eight weeks 90.7% of the pores of the PA cylinder were filled with newly synthesized calcified bone (Fig. 1). This percentage did not essentially change up to 52 weeks after implantation of the cylinder. At the same time, clear breakdown of PA was mea-

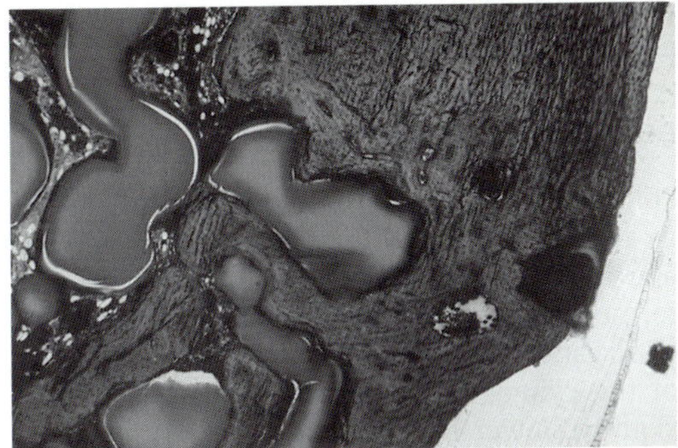

Fig. 1 Microphotograph of the cortical defect in the proximal part of the femur filled with the Polyactive cylinder. The pores in between the Polyactive parts, recognized as the evenly stained parts on this photograph, are almost fully filled with dense bone, over the whole depth of the defect.

sured using the Quantimet analysis, while intimate bone-PA contact remained present (Fig. 2). The control side in the femoral cortex (left, untreated defect) showed only marginal bone formation, even 52 weeks after the operation.

In the bone marrow of the femur the PA cylinders were predominantly filled with bone marrow cells and some connective tissue. At four weeks only 10.4% of the pores were filled with bone while this percentage decreased signifi-

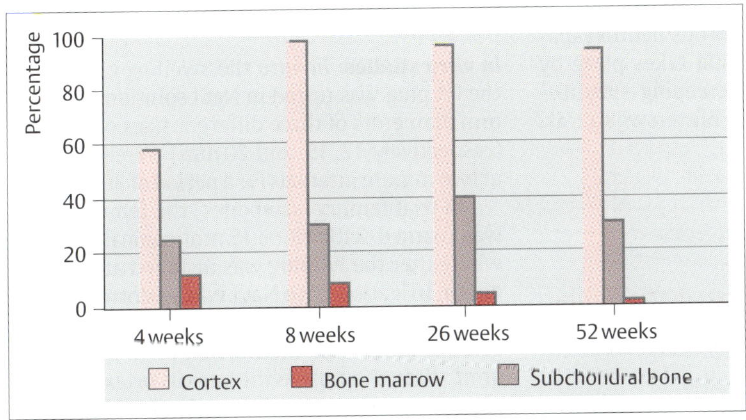

Fig. 2 Percentage of the pores filled with bone 4, 8, 26, and 52 weeks after implantation. Already after 8 weeks approximately 95% of the pores is fully filled with bone in the cortical zone of the defect. In the subchondral defect in the knee, a maximum of 40% of the pores was filled with reduced to about 30% 52 weeks after implantation. This percentage is in accordance with the extent of bone normally present in the subchondral region. In the bone marrow hardly any bone has been formed 26 and 52 weeks after the operation.

cantly to 2.6% and below 1% after respectively eight and twenty-six weeks.

Discussion

Polyactive cylinders 70/30 and 60/40 were tested as a bone graft substitute in a rabbit model. Image analysis of histological sections was performed on samples obtained at four, eight, twenty-six, and fifty-two weeks after the implantation of the cylinders. PA 60/40 cylinders showed a slightly slower bone formation than the 70/30 cylinders, allthough from 26 weeks onwards the total amount of bone present proved to be the same for both. The results suggest that bone formation in the presence of PA followed Wolff's law of bone architecture: the structure in bone is the result of a dynamic regulatory process controlled by mechanical loads (Wolff, 1892). Bone formation in this study occurred depending on the direction and the amount of stress induced in the bone, thereby showing that, in dependence on the location, different amounts of bone were formed in time (Fig. **3**). Bone formation occurred from the edges of the PA cylinder on inwards towards the center. This was found both in the cortex as well as in the trabecular bone. These results are indicative for the bone-bonding property of PA (Bakker et al., 1990; Blitterswijk et al., 1992; Frost et al., 1983; Radder, 1994). As compared to other bone graft substitutes such as demineralized bone matrix or coral, PA has the specific property of new bone formation even in the center. This is in contrast to porous hydroxyapatite (HA), where bone formation takes place by slow and limited peripheral creeping substitution (Blitterswijk et al., 1985; Blitterswijk et al., 1987; Holmes et al., 1987).

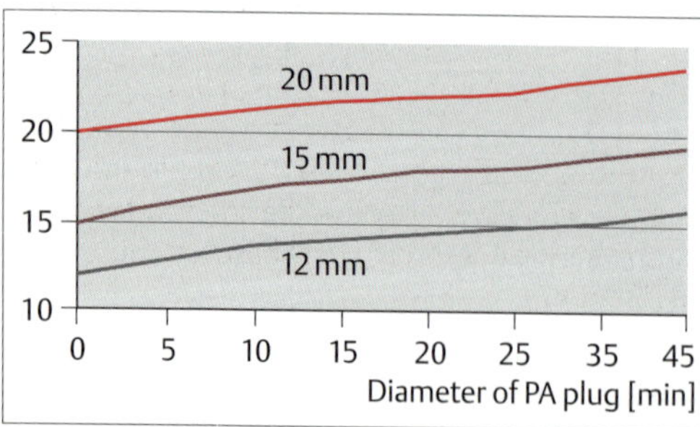

Fig. **3**   Swelling of the PA plug in NaCl, showing an important increase in the bottom diameter of the PA plug in the presence of NaCl, already 10 minutes after installation of the plug.

In contrast to HA, PA has no primary mechanical stability. However, after 8 weeks all the pores of PA are almost completely filled with interconnected bone, that is supposed to have a good mechanical stability. In contrast to HA, PA is very easy to manipulate in the operating room. In conclusion it can be stated that Polyactive is a suitable substitute for auto- or allografts. It is bioerodible, fully biocompatible, and moreover bioactive, stimulating new bone formation without the ned of additives.

Assessment of the Quality of Occlusion of the Femoral Canal with a PA Cement Retainer

Because of the differential properties of PA we decided to develop a new cement retainer. The reason for this development was that in about 25% of our hips the polyethylene Thackray retainer that we used failed due to leakage past the plug, distal migration of the plug, and breaking of parts of the plug during installation in the femoral canal.

In an *in vitro* study in bones, the retention power, the migration, and leakage along a newly designed, conically-shaped elastomeric and degradable cement plug were evaluated. Later on in a pilot study in patients receiving a total hip replacement for osteoarthrosis, the new PA cement retainer was tested (Bulstra, 1996).

Materials and Methods

In vitro **studies:** *In vitro* the swelling capacity of the PA plug was tested in NaCl solution. The bottom diameters of three different sizes of the plug (respectively 12, 15, and 20 mm) were measured at two minute intervals for a period of 30 minutes.

In trial femurs (sawbones) the femoral canal was reamed with 13 or 15 mm conical reamers, whereafter the PA plug was installed at a certain depth. Irrigation with NaCl was performed for 10 minutes in all the cases. Pressures just above the cement plug were measured over a water column, through a hole in the lateral cortex of the femur. The pressure canulla was fixed with glue airtight in the femur.

A cement gun was used to apply the cement after having been cemented in the proximal femur. In this way a secure lock was created in the proximal femur. Cement was then applied using hand force, and maximum pressure was maintained during hardening of the cement.

Table **1**   Cementation pressures and leakage past the PA, respectively, the Thackray plug. Pressures are given in KPa, leakage is shown by + or –. Results show a statistically important difference in the reached intramedullary pressures and the extent of leakage in favor of the PA plug

Plug type	PA 10 mm	PA 12 mm	PA 15 mm	Thackray
13 mm reamer	18.6 (+)	18.6 (±)	21.3 (–)	2 (++)
16 mm reamer	9.3 (+)	18.6 (±)	18.6 (±)	2 (++)

Results *in vitro* Studies

The swelling capacity of the PA plug proved to be considerable (Fig. **3**, Fig. **4**). Already after 10 minutes the bottom diameter of the plugs had increased by 15% or more. The cementation pressures reached for the different sizes of the plug compared to the Thackray plug are shown in Table **1**. Maximum pressures reached are significantly higher in the cases where the PA plug was used even when an undersized plug was installed. Leakage past the plug or distal migration of the plug under the influence of the cementation pressure occurred in a significantly lower percentage in the PA plug cases than in those of the Thackray plug.

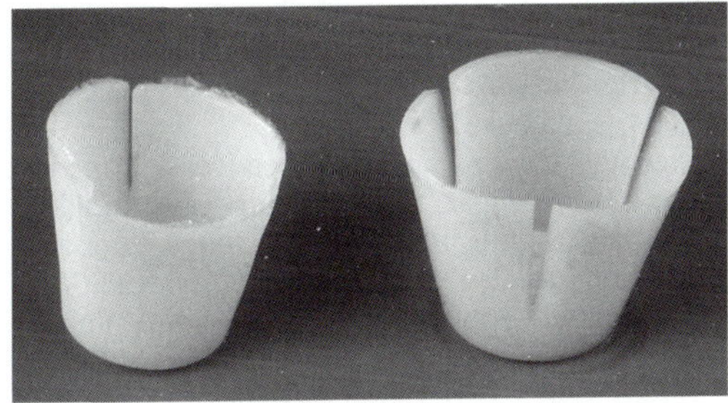

Fig. **4**   Photograph of the PA plug, left prior to installation in NaCl, right 10 minutes after installation on NaCl.

Conclusion *in vitro* Studies

From these *in vitro* studies we learned that the PA plug ensured secure closure of the distal femoral canal during cementation, with much higher cementation pressures than we could reach with the Thackray plug. We supposed that not only the chosen form for the plug but also the swelling properties of the hydrogel are responsible for the good fit of the plug inside the irregular femoral canal.

Clinical Pilot Study

Encouraged by the above-mentioned results, we decided to perform a pilot study in patients receiving a cemented total hip prosthesis for osteoarthritis.

Material and Methods

Twenty-one patients were included with informed consent for the *in vivo* feasability study of the PA plug. The pelvis and the operated femur were X-rayed before and directly after the operation, and X-rays were repeated 3, 6, 12, and 24 months after the operation. During the operation the depth of placement of the PA plug was measured and recorded.

The operation technique included that always first the femoral side was prepared and the PA plug was installed. Before installation of the plug the antero-posterior and the latero-medial diameter of the femoral canal was assessed with a specially developed measuring device. The smallest diameter was chosen for the sizing of the PA plug.

Thereafter, irrigation with NaCl was performed and the acetabular side was prepared.

Clinically, the patients were followed up using the modified Harris hip score for two years. The position of the plug was assessed on the postoperative X-rays and compared to the position of implantation during the operation. Also the extent of leakage of cement was recorded on the post-operative X-rays, while attention was given to the local femoral shaft bone at the site of the PA plug.

Results

All 21 patients with a follow-up of at least two years could be included in the study. In two patients migration of or leakage past the PA plug was observed. In all other patients no migration

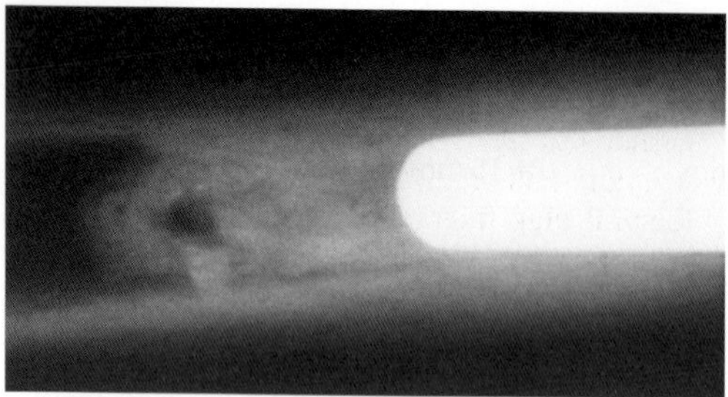

Fig. 5 Photograph of X-ray, showing the distal cement just proximal to the PA plug, one year after implantation of the plug. No cement leakage, or local bone changes are observed.

or leakage was observed (Fig. 5). Clinically, the patients did not differ from a matched group of patients receiving the Thackray cement plug. With a minimum of two years follow-up local changes of the bone at the site of the PA plug were never observed.

Discussion

In the two cases where leakage or migration was observed we found a considerable mismatch in the diameter of the femoral canal at the site of the plug. The antero-posterior diameter of the femoral canal proved to be much larger than the latero-medial diameter in these cases. We suppose that in these cases we should have chosen the largest diameter for the PA plug instead of the smallest as we did in this study.

We conclude that the PA plug proved to be an efficient and safe tool for the occlusion of the femoral canal during cementation. In a future prospective study the largest size of the femoral canal should be used in assessing the best size for the PA plug.

Acknowlegement

The authors would like to express their gratitude to Miss A. Meetens who was responsible for all the data collection and computer assistance necessary to perform these studies.

References

Amstutz HC, Markolf KL, McNeice GN, Green DA. Loosening of total hip replacement components, cause and prevention. In The Hip 1976; Proceedings of the fourth open scientific meeting of the hip society, 102–116, St. Louis, C.V. Mosby.

Ashok SP, Hodgkinson JP. A new femoral cement restrictor. J Arthroplasty 1992; 7, supp.: 411–3.

Bakker D, Blitterswijk van CA, Daems WTh, Grote JJ. Biocompatibility of six elastomers *in vitro*. J Biomed Mater Res 1988; 22: 423–39.

Bakker D, Blitterswijk van CA, Hesseling SC, Daems WT, Grote JJ. Tissue/biomaterial interface characteristics of four elastomers. A transmission electron microscopical study. J Biomed Mat Res 1990; 24: 272–93.

Bakker D, Grote JJ, Vrouenraets CMF, Hesseling SC, Wijn de JR, Blitterswijk van CA. Bone-bonding polymer (Polyactive). In: Heimke G, Soltesz U, Lee AJC (eds.). Advances in Biomaterials, 9, Clin Impl Mat London: Elseviers Science Publishers 1990: 99–104.

Beim GM, Lavernia C, Convery FR. Intramedullary plugs in cemented hip arthroplasty. J Arthroplasty 1989; 4: 139–41.

Beumer GJ, Blitterswijk van CA, Ponec M. Degradative behaviour of polymeric matrices in (sub)dermal and muscle tissue of the rat: a quantitative study. Biomater 1994; 15: 551–9.

Beumer GJ, Blitterswijk van CA, Ponec M. Biocompatibility of a degradable matrix used as a skin substitute: an *in vitro* evaluation. J Biomed Mater Res 1994; 28: 545–52.

Blitterswijk van CA, Bakker D, Leenders H, Brink van der J, Hesseling SC, Bovell YP, Radder AM, Sakkers RJ, Gaillard ML, Heinze PH, Beuiner. Interfacial reactions leading to bone-bonding with PEO/PBT copolymers (Polyactive). In: Ducheyne P, Kokubo T, Blitterswijk van CA (eds.). Bone-bonding Biomaterials, Leiderdorp, The Netherlands. Reed Healthcare Communications 1992: 13–30.

Blitterswijk van CA, Brink van der J, Leenders H, Bakker D. The effect of PEO ratio on degradation, calcification and bone bonding with PEO/PBT copolymers (Polyactive). Cell Mater 1993; 3: 23–36.

Blitterswijk van CA, Grote JJ, Hesseling SC, Bakker D. Polyactive: A bone-bonding polymer. In: Williams KR, Toni A, Middleton J, Palotti G (eds.). Interfaces in medicine and Mechanics-2, Vol. 2. London: Elsevier Science Publishers, a: 1991: 1–9.

Blitterswijk van CA, Grote JJ, Kuijpers W, Blokvan Hoek CJG, Daems WT. Bioreactions at the tissue/hydroxyapatite interface. Biomaterials 1985: 6: 243–51

Blitterswijk van CA, Grote JJ, Kuijpers W, Daems WT, Groot de K. Macropore tissue ingrowth: a quantitative and qualitative study on hydroxyapatite ceramic. Biomaterials 1986; 7: 137–43.

Bucholz RW, Carlton A, Holmes RE. Hydroxyapatite and tricalcium phosphate bone graft substitutes. Orthop Clin North Amer 1987; 18: 323–34.

Bulstra SK, Geesink RGT, Bakker DJ, Bulstra TH, Bouwmeester SJM, van der Linden AJ. *In vitro* and *in vivo* assessment of the quality of occlusion of the femoral canal with a novel resorbable and flexible cementplug. J Bone Joint Surg 1996; 78-B: 892–99.

Bulstra SK, Kuijer R, Blitterswijk van CA, Bulstra TH, Linden van der AJ. Bone formation in Polyactive plugs in the rabbit femur. Orthopedic Research Society, February 1994, New Orleans.

Frost HM. Grafting material observed radiographically for a period of three years. J Oral Implantol 1990; 16: 173–82.

Geesink RGT. Hydroxyl-apatite coated implants: experimental and clinical studies. In: Ducheyne P, Kokubo T, Blitterswijk van CA (eds.). Bone-bonding Biomaterials, Leiderdorp, The Netherlands. Reed healthcare Communications 1992: 121–38.

Grote JJ, Bakker D, Hesseling SC, Blitterswijk van CA. New alloplastic tympanic membrane material. Amer J Otology 1991; 12: 329–35.

Harris WH, McCarthy JC, O'Neill DA. Femoral component loosening using contemporary techniques of femoral cement fixation. J Bone and Joint Surg 1982; 64-A: 1063–7.

Holmes RE, Bucholz RW, Mooney V. Porous hydroxyapatite as a bone graft substitute in diaphyseal defects: a histometric study. J Orthop Res 1987; 5: 114–21.

Huiskes R, Nunamaker D. Local stresses and bone adaptation around orthopaedic implants. Calcif Tissue Int 1984; 36: 110–7.

Johnson JA, Johnson D, Hawary RE, Tan SR, Wong LA, Gross M. Occlusion and stability of synthetic femoral canal plugs used in cemented hip arthroplasty. J Applied Biomat 1995; 6: 213–8.

Kristiansen B, Jensen JS. Biomechanical factors in loosening of the Stanmore hip. Acta Orthop Scand 1985; 56: 21.

Lindberg HO, Carlsson AS. Mechanical loosening of the femoral component in total hip replacement: Brunswik design. Acta Orthop Scand 1983; 54: 557.

Loon van JA. Tissue reactions during long term implantation in relation to degradation. A study of a range of PEO/PBT copolymers; Abstract 20 th Annual Meeting of the society for biomaterials 1994; April 5–9, Boston, Ma, USA.

Mallory TH. A plastic intermedullary plug for total hip arthroplasty. Clin Orthop Rel Res 1981; 155: 37–40.

Muschler GF, Huber B, Ullman T, Barth R, Easly K, Otis JO, Lane JM. Evaluation of bone-grafting materials in a new canine segmental spinal fusion model. J Orthop Res 1993; 11: 514–24.

Northmore-Ball MD, Narang OV, Vergroesen D. Distal femoral plug migration with cement pressurization in revision surgery and a simple technique for its prevention. J Arthroplasty, Sept. 1991; 6: 199–201.

Oh I, Carlson CE, Tomford WW, Haris WH. Improved fixation of the femoral component after total hip replacement using a methacrylate intramedullary plug. J Bone and Joint Surg 1987; 60-A: 608–13.

Osborn JF, Newesly H. Dynamic aspects of the implants bone interface. In Dental Implants. Carl Hansen Verlag, Munich, Germany 1980; 111–23.

Radder AM. Bone bonding copolymers for hard tissue replacement. Thesis 1995; University of Leiden, The Netherlands.

Radder AM, Leenders H, Blitterswijk van CA. Interface reactions to PEO/PBT copolymers (Polyactive): A study on bone bonding. J Biomed Mater Res 1994; 28: 141–51.

Radder AM. Bone-bonding copolymers for hard tissue replacement, Ph. D. Thesis, Leiden, 1994.

Sakkers RJB. Relation between swelling pressure of PEO-PBT copolymers and bursting pressure of human femoral bones. In: Doherty PJ et al. (eds.). Advances in biomaterials. Elsevier Science Publishers 1992; 357–61.

Shalaby SW, Burg KJL. Bioabsorbable polymers update: degradation mechanisms, safety and application. J Applied Biomat 1995; 6: 219–21.

Thomsen NOB, Jensen TT, Uhrbrand B, Mossing NB. Intramedullary plugs in total hip arthroplasty. J Arthroplasty 1992; 7, supp.: 415–8.

Wenda K, Degreif J, Runkel M, Ritter G. Pathogenesis and prophylaxis of circulatory reactions during total hip replacement. Arch Orthop Trauma Surg 1993; 112: 260–5.

Wheelwright EF, Byrick RJ, Wigglesworth DF. Hypotension during cemented arthroplasty, relationship to cardiac output and fat embolism. J Bone J Surg 1993; 75 B: 715–23.

Wolff J. Das Gesetz der Transformation der Knochen. Hirschwald, Berlin 1892.

Development of a Biodegradable Wound Covering and First Clinical Results

Ch. Jürgens, H.-R. Kricheldorf, I. Kreiser-Saunders

Introduction

In the last 20 years, many synthetic materials have been developed for use as wound dressings for large area burns or split-skin donor sites. Their essential advantage over textile coverings or fatty gauze is their impermeability to germs and a reduction of water loss.

Whereas in other areas of surgery, synthetic absorbable materials have found a firm place as sutures, tissue padding, clips, or bone pins (Langer, 1993; Pitt, 1981; Vainionpää, 1989), there are still very few publications on the use of such materials as dressings (Gogolewski, 1983; Jürgens, 1995). The objective of using degradable dressings is to avoid changing dressings with the associated retraumatization of the wound and pain for the patient. Other advantages lie in the possibility of the simultaneous use of the dressing as a drug delivery system, since integration and controlled release of pharmacologically active substances is possible in principle (Hutchinson, 1987; Wise, 1979). However, an effect on the wound healing can be expected due to the degradation products released during degradation.

Chemical Development

Polylactide and polycaprolactone have proved useful as degradable materials for various medical applications because of their good biocompatibility (Pitt, 1981; Vainionpää, 1989; Wise, 1979). Because of this good tolerability, D,L-lactide and ε-caprolactone were selected for synthesis. The hydrolytic degradation of the polymers releases 6-hydroxycaproic acid and lactic acid which are metabolized *in vivo* via β-oxidation as acetyl-CoA or broken down in the lactic acid cycle.

The physical properties and degradation behavior of lactide-caprolactone copolymers are far more variable than those of homopolymers, and can be affected by the monomer-initiator ratio, the polymerization temperature and dura-

tion, and the quantity ratio of the monomers. The material is amorphous and thermoplastic.

One hundred and fifty different copolymers have been produced and characterized with the established methods of chemical analysis. GPC and viscosimetry are important for assessing the molecule chain length and are used to study the degradation behavior under hydrolysis. DSC determines the range of the softening temperature (glass transition temperature, T_G) of thermoplastics. Below this temperature, the polymers are hard and fragile and only become soft and plastic when T_G is reached. Therefore at body temperature, copolymers with a T_G below 25 °C become very soft and vulnerable and would stick to textiles. If the softening temperature is set above 37 °C, the material remains hard and inflexible at skin temperature and cannot adapt to the skin surface. Polymers to be used as dressings must therefore be made with a T_G of between 25 °C and 37 °C. Nuclear spin spectroscopy is used for sequence analysis, and densitometry to establish the specific density.

Methods

In parallel to the chemical development, *in vitro* tests were carried out to select suitable polymers for animal tests and clinical use in view of their physical properties. Three copolymers were selected with the following characteristics (Table 1).

Table 1 Physical properties of copolymers C308, C309 and C310.

Property	Polymer		
	C308	C309	C310
Elution volume V_e (ml)	24.45	25.78	26.52
Glass temperature T_G (°C)	31.29	24.9	36.42
Viscosity (dl/g)	0.621	0.492	0.7681
Density (g/cm³)	1.236	1.23	1.24

Sheets 20–40 μm thick were produced from these polymers. Polymer C310 was made microporous in structure by a hygroscopic additive. The γ-sterilized sheet material was tested for structure, transparency, mechanical strength, water vapor permeability, and the surface pH value and compared with three conventional dressings made of polyurethane (Tegaderm™, Omiderm™, and Opsite™). Changes under hydrolysis were established for the absorbable sheets on the 2nd, 5 th, 10 th, and 15 th day after exposure in water. A few methods and results will be shown here.

Water Vapor Permeability

The water vapor permeation through sheets depends on the material, the thickness, the temperature, relative humidity, and air flow. Whereas material properties, temperature, and relative humidity can be defined or measured, the flow speed of the air under clinical conditions is difficult to assess. Therefore measurements of water vapor permeability were carried out in two different methods with flow speeds of approximately 1.0 l/min (ventilated chamber) and 0.0 l/min (Evaporimeter EP1. Servomed AB, Stockholm), which led to comparable results (Jürgens, 1995).

Surface pH-Measurements

The hydrolysis of the copolymers into lactic acid and 6-hydroxycaproic acid in an aqueous environment will lead to a reduction in the pH value. These pH value changes were recorded with a pH surface measurement probe (Hamilton, Switzerland) and a pH meter (WTW, Weinheim).

After the test of the chemical and physical properties of copolymer sheets of D,L-lactide and ε-caprolactone, the suitability of the material as a dressing for clinical use was tested by toxicological and bacteriological tests *in vitro* and in animal tests on the rat.

Toxicological Tests

The cellular and tissue compatibility of polylactide and polycaprolactone has already been proven in several studies and in the American Gentox Program (Sweet, 1987). Therefore the proof of toxicological safety for the copolymers was restricted to the MTT test with HeLa cells (Borenfreund, 1988) and the cultivation of keratinocyte cultures (Rosdy, 1990; Rheinwald, 1975) on the lactide-caprolactone sheets.

Bacteriological Tests

The bacteriological *in vitro* tests were carried out in different test arrangements. The permeability of the sheets to nutrient media, the growth of bacterial colonies beneath the copolymer sheets and the germ permeation time under hydrolysis was tested using cultures of *Staphylococcus aureus, Escherichia coli, Pseudomonas aeruginosa,* and *Enterococcus faecalis.*

In vivo Tests

The *in vivo* tests were carried out on Dark Agouti rats (DA/Han). The application properties and behavior of the sheets on the wound and reactions of the wound base were tested and compared with a reference sheet of polyurethane (Opsite™). Skin and subcutaneous tissue of the back of the anesthetized animals were excised in an externt of 5×7 cm². The dressing sheet samples were applied and attached to the edge of the wound with a continuous suture. The individual test duration was 2, 5, 10, 13, 15, and 18 days.

The pain reactions and behavior of the test animals were observed in particular. The application properties and changes to the dressings on the wound were recorded with regard to adherence and transparency. Bleeding, vascular proliferation, and wound contraction were recorded planimetrically and the retention of wound exudate below the sheets was assessed visually.

Surface pH value measurements of the wound were made in analogy to the *in vitro* studies in order to show changes in the wound environment in comparison with the polyurethane sheet. Biopsies for the histology were taken from the wound edge and the wound centre. Different staining methods were used to color the histological sections.

Clinical Application

On the basis of the results, the application for clinical use and testing on split-skin donor sites was permitted by the Ethics commission. Application, subjective assessment by patients and staff, complications, local hyperemia and temperature loss by thermography and systemic effects by measurement of plasma lactate were evaluated.

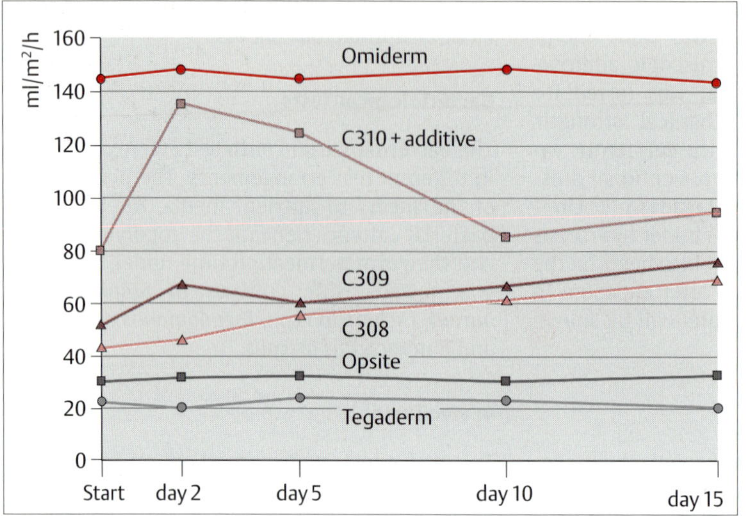

Fig. 1 The water vapor permeation through non-degradable sheets remains constant. The high permeability of the microporous copolymer sheet C310 in the first 5 days and the subsequent reduction is significant.

Results

Water Vapor Permeability

The water vapor permeability of the copolymer films varies as a function of the molecular weight distribution, sheet structure, and additives and increases under hydrolysis. Microporous sheets (C310) are essentially more permeable than the solid film sheets (C308, C309) (Fig. 1). A considerable increase in permeation was established in the first 5 days. From the fifth day, the vapor permeability decreases again corresponding to the lower wound exudation. On the basis of these changes in water vapor permeation, microporous copolymer sheets are the most suitable of the sheets tested for controlled fluid loss. The dressings with adhesive layer (Tegaderm™, Opsite™) are the least permeable of all materials tested, while Omiderm™ shows the highest water vapor permeability (145 ml/m²/h).

pH Measurements

The pH measurements on the sheet surface *in vitro* show a change from 5.4 to values down to 3.6. As expected, the *in vivo* pH value measurements on the wound base under the sheets showed also a clear shift towards the acid environment compared to the Opsite™ film (Fig. 2).

Cytotoxicity Tests

In the MTT test with the direct contact and the extraction method no toxic effect of the lactide-caprotactone copolymer was seen. The cultivation of keratinocytes on the copolymer sheet showed a confluent epithelial layer after 6 days (Fig. 3). The proliferation was not delayed or deteriorated in comparison with the standard sample, but appeared slightly accelerated.

Bacteriological Tests

The bacterial colonies showed a markedly slower growth on agar plates underneath the copolymer film than colonies beside the film sheet or under Opsite™. Pemeability for bacteria *in vitro* under degradation by hydrolysis was seen at the earliest between the 8 th day (film thickness 25 µ) and the 15 th day (film thickness 35 µ).

In vivo Tests

During the test period, the animals showed no unusual behavior. At no time was their mobility restricted. No pain reactions were observed either with the sheets in place or when the sheet was touched or removed. The dressing was adapted very well to the wound surface on application (Fig. 4a). Due to wound contraction, a folding of the sheets with a fibrin precipitate below the dressings was seen (Fig. 4b). Nevertheless, the wound base could still be assessed well, and

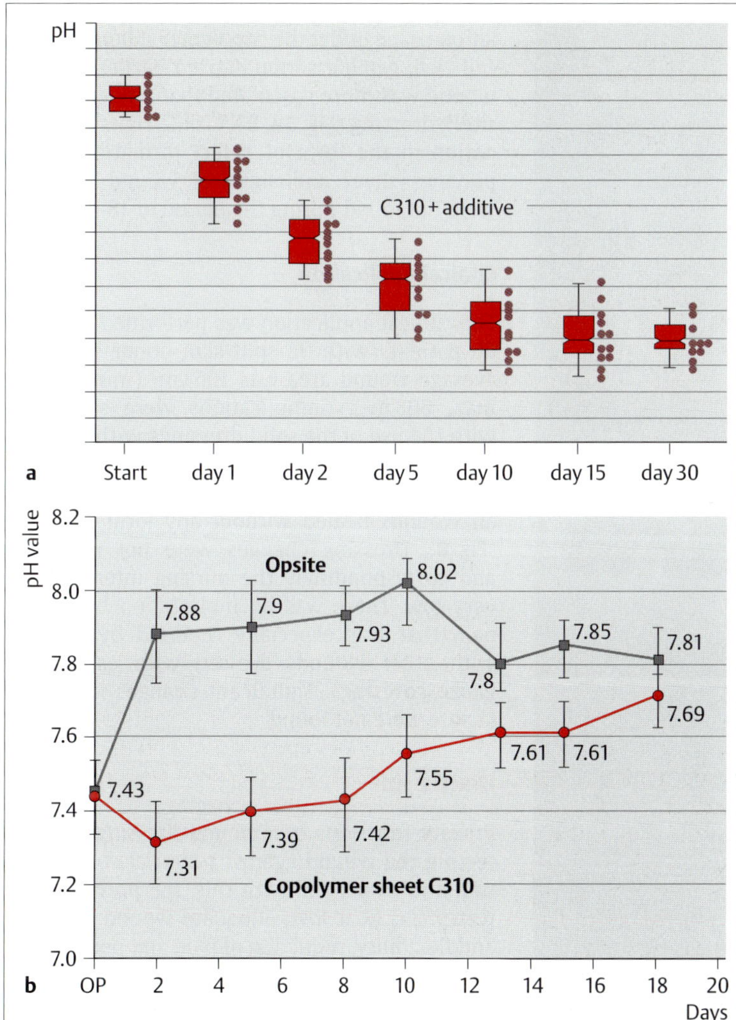

Fig. 2 The surface pH value of the copolymer sheet C310 over time under hydrolysis (**a**) and changes of the pH value of the wound base beneath Opsite™ and the copolymer dressing (**b**).

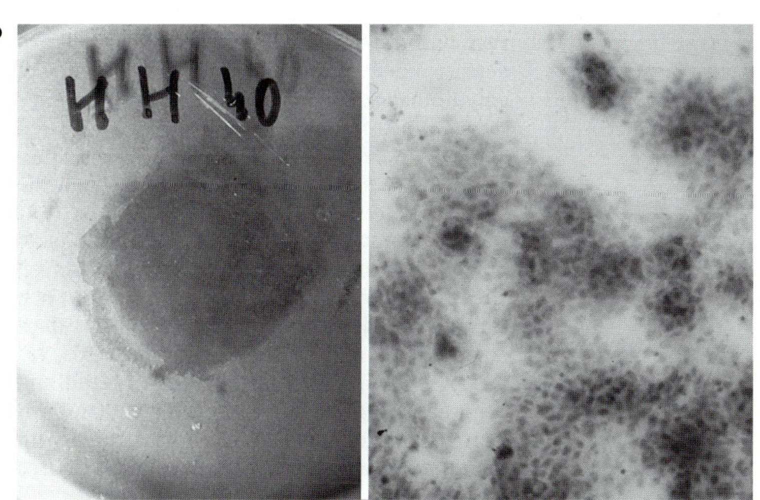

Fig. 3 Confluent epithelial layer of the keratinocytes on top of the copolymer sheet after six days. (**a**) Staining of sample with crystal violet, (**b**) sample with toluidine blue.

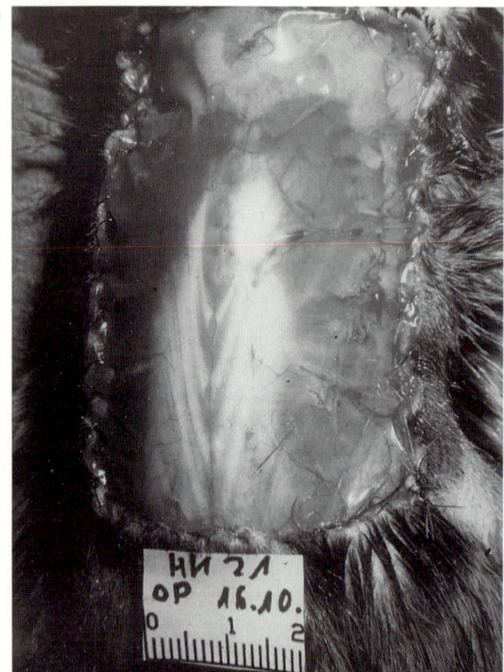

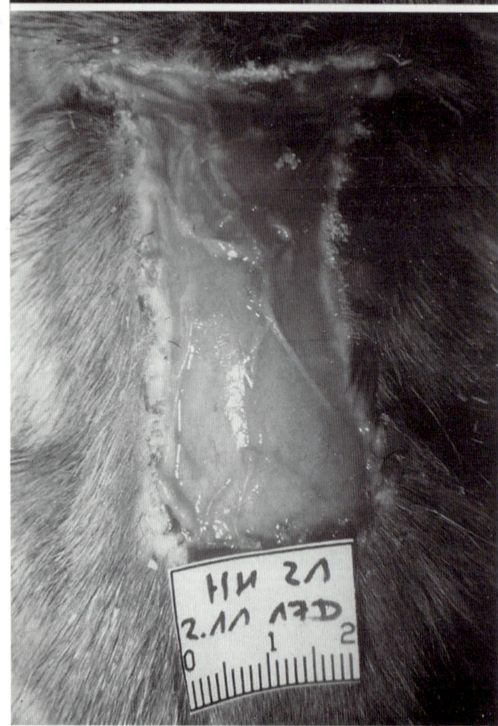

Fig. 4   (a) Copolymer dressing on application with good adherence to the wound surface. (b) After 17 days wound contraction led to a folding of the dressing with fibrin clotting beneath.

new vessels could be clearly detected. The granulation tissue under the copolymer sheets was less cell-rich, capillarization started earlier, and the wound was more vasculated than under the Opsite™ dressing (Fig. **5a, b**). Visible signs of degradation in the form of defect formation in the polymer sheet and signs of wound infection were not found during the period of 18 days.

Clinical Application

The clinical application was performed so far on 60 patients with 62 split-skin donor sites. The average wound area was 105 cm² (min. 20 cm², max. 608 m²). Complications were seen only with the use of the solid dressings with low permeability: leakage in eight cases and three local infections. With the use of the microporous films all wounds healed without any local irritation (Fig. **6**). Dressing changes were not necessary and correspondingly the nursing intensity was very low. There was no molestation by wound pain that was especially reported by patients with other wounds dressed with usual fatty gauze coverings. Significant changes in plasma lactate were not found.

Discussion

Priority functions of a wound dressing are protecting the wound against bacterial contamination and associated with this, the prevention of water and heat loss, adequate wound adhesion and flexibility, reduction of pain and possibly the ability to assess the wound base. These requirements can only be fulfilled by a complete and perfect covering of the wound. The transparency of the copolymer sheets allows the assessment of very fine structures which are clearly harder to detect under the comparison sheets made of polyurethane. Restrictions in the transparency through micropores were deliberately increased with this material to achieve better wound adhesion and water vapor permeability through the structuring.

The water loss via intact skin and skin wounds has been extensively studied (Lamke, 1977). Whereas approximately 200 ml/m²/24 h water evaporate through healthy skin, for third degree burns and split-skin donor wounds, values of 3400–3600 ml/m²/24 h are achieved, and for granulating wounds even over 5000 ml/m²/24 h. A considerable heat loss is associated with the excess evaporation of fluid from large area

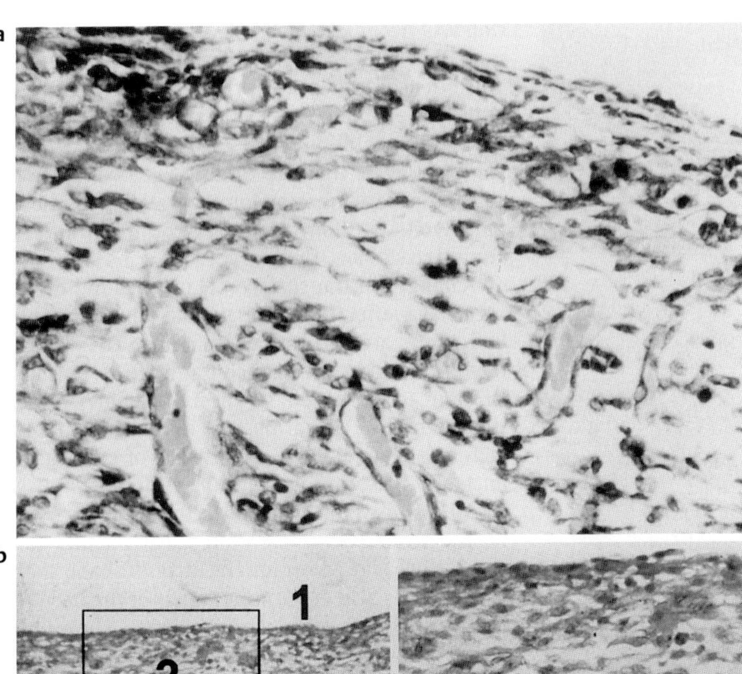

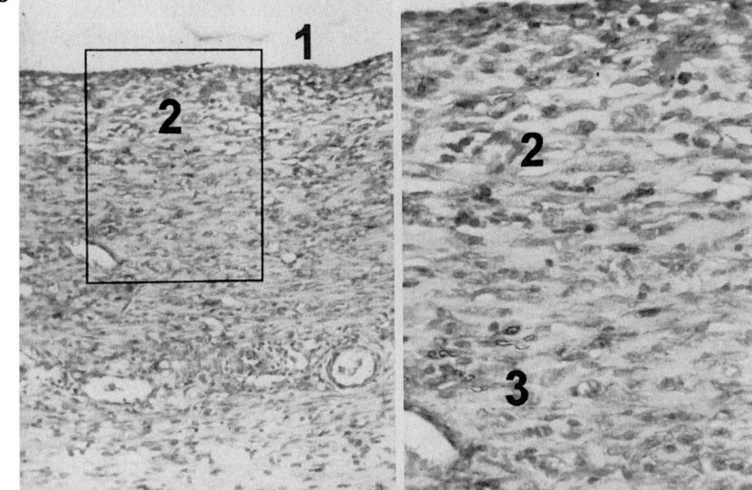

Fig. 5 (**a**) Early capillarization from the wound base to the surface (Giemsa, 400 : 1). (**b**) Granulation tissue with superficial fibroblast layer (1), good vascularization (2), and some polymer fragments (3), without foreign body reaction (hematoxylin-eosin, 100 : 1 and 400 : 1).

wounds. Control of the fluid loss through wound dressing is therefore very important in the treatment of extensive wound areas, in particular in burns. Fluid-permeable dressings do not protect against bacterial contamination, fluid and heat loss and encourage the drying of the wounds. Impermeable materials lead to a retention of wound exudate, therefore causing maceration of the adjacent uninjured integument and mobilization of the local germs. A dressing impermeable to fluids but with a water vapor permeability which is initially high but falls with the reduction in wound exudate, is therefore desirable. The values measured with the evaporimeter for the dressings Te-gaderm™, Opsite™, and Omiderm™ correspond to the data in the literature (Erasmus, 1989; Queen, 1987). The values for the lactide-caprolactone sheets are dependent on the polymer chain length and structure. The water vapor permeation is less with long-chain polymers and increases only slowly in view of the longer degradation times compared with short-chain microporous polymers. The cause of the clear rise in permeability of the microporous sheets during the first days is presumably the hygroscopic additive. The reduction in vapor permeability from the 5 th day can be explained by the wash out of the additive and the predominance of the hydrophobic poly-

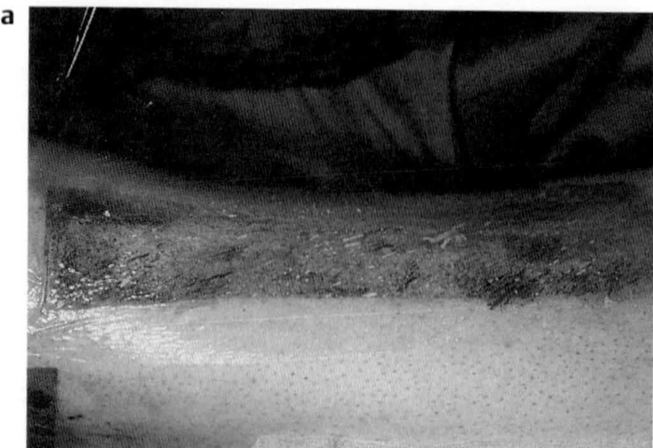

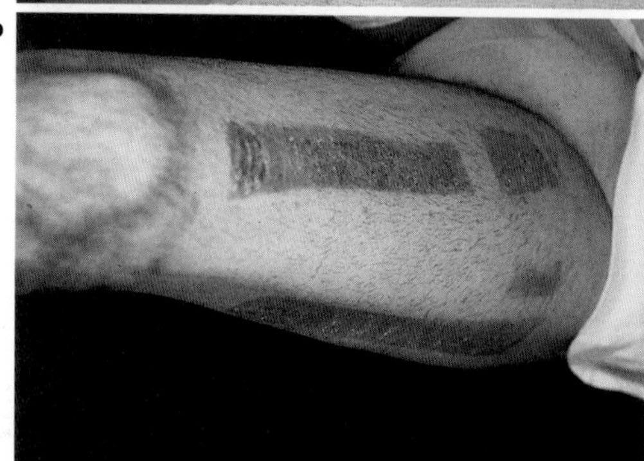

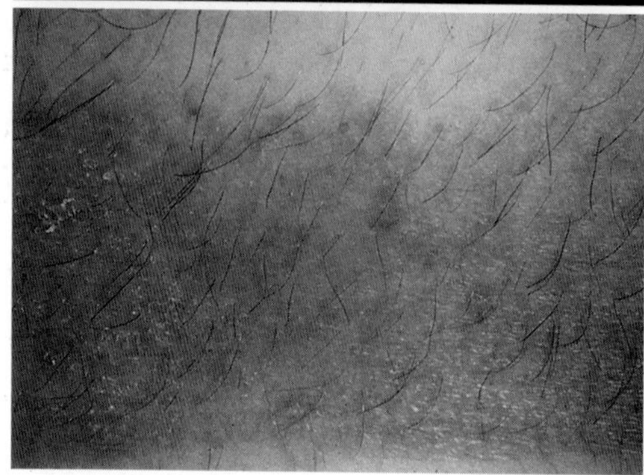

Fig. 6 (a) Application of the copolymer dressing on a split-skin donor site. (b) After 14 days the wound is almost healed with little remainder of the film. (c) Two weeks later one can see reduction of redness and only small fragments of the dressing on the skin.

mer properties. The same effect to a lesser extent may be caused by the hydrophilic monomer components in short-chain polymers. On the basis of these changes in water vapor permeation, microporous sheets are the most suitable of the lactide-caprolactone sheets tested for controlled fluid loss. Because of the very low permeability, it is expected that a considerable exudate reten-

tion will occur with the use of the other copolymer sheets with heavily discharging wounds. This effect is known with the use of Tegaderm™ and Opsite™. Omiderm™ has the highest water vapor permeability of the dressings tested. The values indicate that this dressing is ideal for use as a temporary dressing for very heavily discharging wounds. Clinical studies confirm this assumption (Behar, 1986).

Changes in the surface pH of a wound dressing have effects on the wound environment, and there are indications that low pH values have a favorable effect on contamination, epithelization and collagen synthesis (Kemble, 1975; Wiseman, 1992). Hydrolysis of the lactide-caprolactone sheets leads to the release of lactic acid and 6-hydroxycaproic acid. *In vitro* and *in vivo*, the pH value of the sheet surface and, respectively, the wound base therefore clearly shifts towards the acid environment. It is probably because of this acid environment that in the bacteriological studies the bacterial colonies showed a markedly slower growth underneath the copolymer film. The tests also showed an impermeability of the sheets for germs from the surface of the sheet to the culture medium for a period of at least 15 days. It can therefore be assumed that the germ permeation times under clinical conditions will be essentially delayed and the sheets will guarantee sufficient protection of the wound to secondary contamination.

As expected, the toxicological tests on the copolymers could show that no harmful cytotoxic effects are to be expected when these substances are used as wound dressings. The keratinocyte culture on the copolymer sheet in comparison with the standard sample rather suggests a positive effect on the cell growth, which has been confirmed by other investigators (Reif, 1992, 1994; Soehnchen, 1992).

The advantages of occlusive or semiocclusive wound dressings with regard to wound healing, mobility and pain in comparison with wound treatment with textile dressings or fatty gauze have been extensively demonstrated in the last 30 years (Hutchinson, 1989; James, 1975; Winter, 1962). So in the animal tests as well as in the clinical application, despite the extensive wounds, the freedom of mobility was not affected nor any pain perceived. A retention of wound exudate was particularly clear under Opsite™ but also under the solid copolymer sheets C308 and C309. In contrast, under the microporous sheets, the wound environment was always moist without affecting the adherence to the wound base. In the histological tests, only slight differences in wound healing could be found under Opsite™ and the copolymer sheets. The granulation tissue under the lactide-caprolactone sheets was less cell-rich and more vasculated. A faster epithelization from the wound edge could be assumed but not certainly be proven on the basis of the individual observations.

Conclusions

There are at least two reasons for the use of a biodegradable wound dressing:

1. *No dressing changes:* with a decrease of secondary wound contamination and nursing intensity and an increase of patients comfort.
2. *The influence on wound healing:* The unspecific influence provided by moist wound environment, water vapor permeability and impermeability for bacteria can also be obtained by other non-degradable dressings. But the specific influence resulting from an acid environment, high local lactate concentration, and a variable vapor permeability can only be achieved by a degradable dressing.

References

Behar D, Juszynski M, Ben Hur N, Golan J, Eldad A, Tuchman Y, Sterenberg N, Rudensky B. Omiderm, a new synthetic wound covering: Physical properties and drug permeability studies. J Biomed Mat Res 1986; 20: 731–8.

Borenfreund E, Babich H, Martin-Alguacil N. Comparison of two *in vitro* cytotoxicity assays – The neutral red (NR) and tetrazolium MTT tests. Toxic in vitro 1988; 2: 1–6.

Erasmus ME, Jonkman MF. Water vapour permeance: a meaningful measure for water vapour permeability of wound coverings. Burns 1989; 15: 371–5.

Gogolewski S, Pennings AJ. An artificial skin based on biodegradable mixtures of polylactides and polyurethanes for full-thickness skin wound covering. Makromol Chem Rapid Commun 1983; 4: 675–80.

Hutchinson FG, Furr BJA. Design of biodegradable polymers for controlled release. In: Johnson P, Lloyd-Jones JG (eds.). Drug delivery systems. VCH Verlagsgesellschaft, Weinheim, New York 1987: 106–19.

Hutchinson JJ. Prevalence of wound infection under occlusive dressings: A collective survey of reported research. Wounds 1989; 1: 123–33.

James JH, Watson ACH. The use of Opsite, a vapour permeable dressing, on skin graft donor sites. Brit J Plast Surg 1975; 28: 107–10.

Jürgens Ch, Porte T, Wolter D, Schmidt H, Kricheldorf H, Kreiser-Saunders I. Entwicklung und Charakterisierung einer absorbierbaren temporären Wundabdeckung. Unfallchirurg 1995; 98: 233–40.

Kemble JVH. pH changes on the surface of burns. Brit J Plast Surg 1975; 28: 181–4.

Lamke LO, Nilsson GE, Reithner HL. The evaporative water loss from burns and the water vapour permeability of grafts and artifical membranes used in the treatment of burns. Burns 1977; 3: 159–65.

Langer R, Vacanti JP. Tissue engineering. Science 1993; 260: 920–5.

Pitt CG, Gratzl MM, Kimmel GL, Surles J, Schindler AD. Aliphatic polyesters II. The degradation of poly(DL-lactide), poly(ε-caprolactone), and their copolymers *in vivo*. Biomaterials 1981; 2: 215–20.

Queen D, Gaylor JDS, Evans JH, Courtney JM. The preclinical evaluation of the water vapour transmission rate through burn wound dressings. Biomaterials 1987; 8: 367–71.

Reif K. Personal communications. Pharmatec, Frankfurt, 1992, 1994.

Rheinwald JG, Green H. Serial cultivation of strains of human epidermal keratinocytes: The formation of keratinizing colonies from single cells. Cell 1975; 6: 331–44.

Rosdy M, Clauss LC. Cytotoxicity testing of wound dressings using normal human keratinocytes in culture. J Biomed Mat Res 1990; 24: 363–77.

Soehnchen R, Jürgens Ch, Daniels H, Hilbert E, Orfanos C. Biodegradierbare Polymere als Trägermatrix für kultivierte Keratinozyten. Abstract: 15. Jahrestagung der Vereinigung für operative und onkologische Dermatologie, Köln, 1992.

Sweet DV. Registry of toxic effects of chemical substances. US Department of Health and Human Services, Public Health Service, 1985–86 Edition, 1987.

Vainionpää S, Rokkanen P, Törmälä P. Surgical applications of biodegradable polymers in human tissues. Prog Polym Sci 1989; 14: 679–716.

Winter GD. Formation of the scab and the rate of epithelialisation of superficial wounds in the skin of the young domestic pig. Nature 1962; 193: 293–4.

Wise DL, Fellmann TD, Sanderson JE, Wentworth RL. Lactic/Glycolic Acid Polymers. In: Gregoriadis G. (ed.). Drug carriers in Biology and Medicine. Academic Press, London, New York, San Francisco, 1979: 237–70.

Wiseman DM, Parm S, Rovee DT, Alvarez OM. Wound dressings: Design and use. In: Cohen IK, Diegelmann RF, Lindblad WJ. (eds.). Wound healing. W. B. Saunders Company, Philadelphia, London, Toronto, Montreal, Sydney, Tokyo, 1992; 563–77.

Bioresorbable Polymers as Drug Delivery Systems

A. Göpferich

Introduction

Polymers are a valuable source of biomaterials. They were first used as non-degradable materials to provide a mechanical function for which the erosion of polymer was highly undesirable. It was soon recognized, however, that polymer degradation could be an advantage for many applications. An obvious benefit, for example, is the circumvention of the post-application removal of a device. One of the first fields taking advantage of biodegradable polymers is surgery. As suture material, screws or plates, degradable polymers provide a mechanical function for a limited period of time (Leenslang, 1987). Nowadays, degradable polymers are also in use for applications during which they contribute directly to success by their degradation and erosion. Examples are the use of degradable polymer scaffolds in tissue engineering for the repair of tissue and organs (Langer and Vacanti, 1993) and erosion-controlled release from degradable polymers in the field of drug delivery (Langer, 1990). Although the latter application stems from pharmaceutics it has also an impact on the area of biomaterials. Degradable polymer scaffolds in tissue engineering, for example, are increasingly intended not only to provide a mechanical support and guidance to growing cells and tissues but also to release sensitive substances such as growth factors safely during an application.

The above-mentioned applications depend markedly on the degradation and erosion properties of polymers. It is, therefore, essential to understand according to which mechanisms erosion and degradation proceed. This is especially true if degradable polymers are intended to be used for the delivery of drugs. Two examples that illustrate why erosion phenomena are important for drug release from degradable polymers are the physical and chemical stability of sensitive drugs such as proteins and peptides and the kinetics of drug release:

– Protein and peptide drugs have been found to be instable at extreme pH values or at high osmotic pressure. Such conditions have been found to exist to some extent during the erosion of biodegradable polymers (Brunner and Göpferich, 1996).
– The need for the controlled release of drugs from eroding polymers is obvious. Implants that are intended to release potent drugs over years carry an enormous dose of drug and one has to make sure that an uncontrolled release cannot occur.

Polymer Degradation and Erosion

Polymer degradation and erosion are important processes for the control of drug release from bioerodible polymers. As different definitions exist in the literature, it is important to define both terms. *Degradation* is the process of polymer chain scission while *erosion* is the mass loss of a polymer matrix (Tamada and Langer, 1993). By virtue of this definition, degradation is part of erosion in the case of a water-insoluble polymer. The loss of molecular weight is a measure for the degradation of a polymer matrix while mass loss is indicative for its erosion. The terms biodegradation and bioerosion imply that biological processes are involved in the overall kinetics. There are 4 types of degradation: chemical, thermal, mechanical, and physical degradation (Göpferich, 1996). For degradable polymers, chemical degradation is the most important mechanism. All biodegradable polymers contain functional groups in their backbone that can be cleaved by hydrolysis. Figure 1 gives a survey on some classes of degradable polymers.

With the help of the definitions above, we should be able to define what a degradable polymer is and how it can be distinguished from non-degradable ones, but in fact we are not. Experiments with ^{14}C labeled polyethylene revealed that also those polymers degrade *in vivo* which

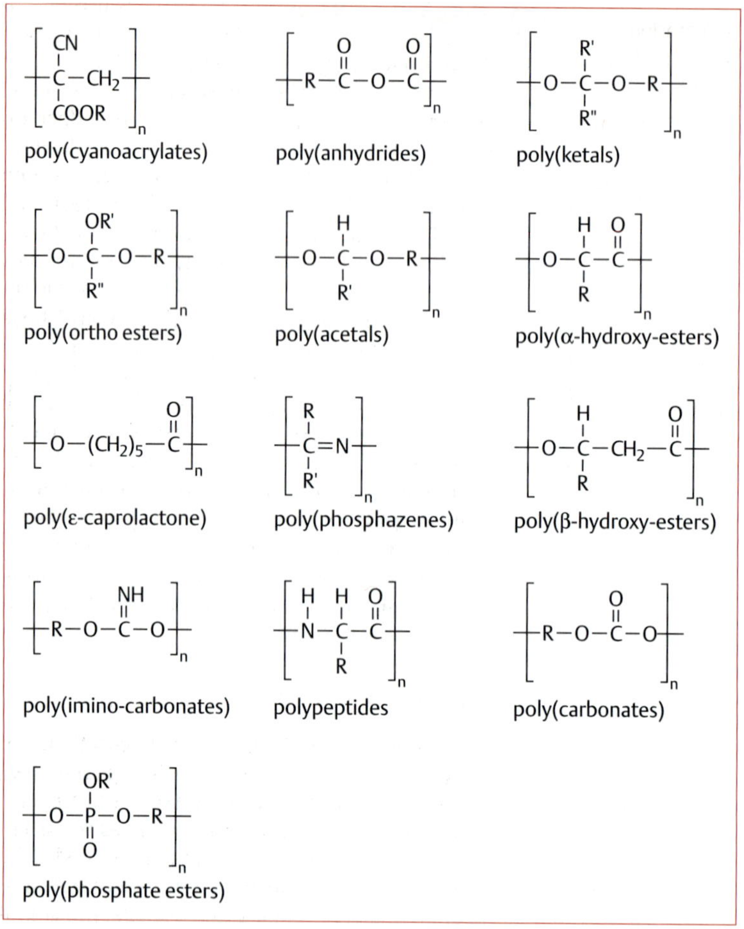

Figure **1** Chemical structures of biodegradable polymers.

poly(cyanoacrylates)　　poly(anhydrides)　　poly(ketals)

poly(ortho esters)　　poly(acetals)　　poly(α-hydroxy-esters)

poly(ε-caprolactone)　　poly(phosphazenes)　　poly(β-hydroxy-esters)

poly(imino-carbonates)　　polypeptides　　poly(carbonates)

poly(phosphate esters)

are usually considered non-degradable (Alberts-son, 1980). Therefore, the potential to degrade cannot be the only criteria to distinguish degradable from non-degradable polymers. An additional criteria is the time scale on which degradation happens. A polymer that does not degrade within the human lifetime is certainly not considered degradable. Therefore dimensionless numbers could be used to define what a degradable polymer is (Göpferich, 1996 b):

$$D = \frac{\text{time of degradation}}{\text{human lifetime}} \qquad (1)$$

Degradable polymers have small values for D (D → 0) and non-degradable polymers have large ones (D → ∞).

The erosion mechanism is an individual characteristic of a polymer and hard to predict based on its formula and a detailed system that allows one to classify degradable polymers according to their erosion mechanism does not exist. However, a crude distinction has been made between bulk eroding and surface eroding polymers. Both mechanisms are illustrated in Figure 2. For a surface eroding polymer matrix, degradation and erosion are so fast that they are confined to the surface while for a bulk eroding polymer, the complete cross section is affected by both processes.

The Release of Drugs from Degradable Polymers

If degradable polymers are intended to be used for the delivery of drugs, the drug release kinetics

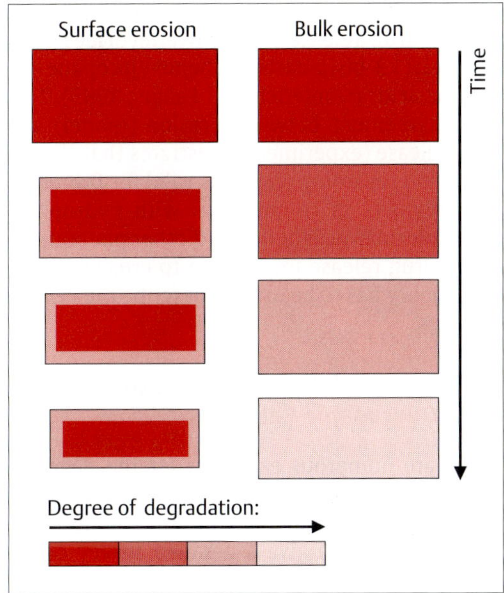

Fig. 2 Schematic illustration of surface erosion and bulk erosion.

are of fundamental importance. On the one hand, the minimum therapeutical concentration has to be established in plasma and tissue while on the other hand toxic concentrations have to be avoided. Therefore, the release of drugs from erodible polymers has to be controlled reliably. For that purpose one can use one of the three major mechanisms of drug release from polymers: diffusion, polymer swelling followed by fast diffusion-controlled release, and polymer erosion. Usually erosion is intended to be the rate controlling mechanism because the complete disappearance of the polymer material coincides with the end of drug release. It is, however, not necessarily only erosion that controls the release of drugs from degradable polymers as it is often assumed. Erosion competes rather with diffusion and polymer swelling. It is obvious that the release of drugs is only purely erosion-controlled if the erosion of polymer is faster than the competing mechanisms. Therefore, one can conclude that fast eroding polymers are good candidates to control drug release by erosion alone. To illustrate the difference in drug release between slow-eroding and fast-eroding polymers, polylactides and polyanhydrides can serve as examples (cf. Figure 1). Both are built from different functional groups. Due to the higher reactivity of the anhy-

dride bond, polyanhydrides have been reported to degrade substantially faster than polylactides. Accordingly, polyanhydrides are mainly surface eroding, while polylactides are bulk eroding polymers. That this has tremendous effect on drug release is revealed when comparing drug release profiles with polymer degradation. When Clenbuterol × HCl was released from extruded poly(D,L-lactic acid) MW 21 000 cylinders, the release profile consisted clearly of two periods (Mayer and Stricker, 1994). Up to 40 days, the release profile was concave which is typical for a system that releases a drug by diffusion. There was no mass loss from the polymer during this period and, therefore, also no erosion. At day 50 the massive release of drug sets in which coincided with the massive erosion of the matrix (Mayer and Stricker, 1994). In the case of drug release from polyanhydride matrices, in contrast, the release coincides with the erosion of the matrix in many cases (Göpferich and Langer, 1995), from which one can conclude that drug release is mainly erosion-controlled.

Polymer Erosion Modeling

To be able to describe polymer erosion theoretically is desirable in many ways. The goal in drug delivery is to find a correlation between the erosion of a carrier material and the release of drugs. There have been only few attempts to model the erosion of degradable polymers. One of the most promising approaches is to model the erosion of polymers using 2 dimensional discrete grids (Göpferich and Langer, 1993; Zygourakis, 1989). Using such methods, the cross section through a matrix is first covered by a rectangular computational grid. This divides a polymer matrix cross section into a multitude of small pieces, so-called pixels. To simulate erosion, the pixels are removed from the grid according to an algorithm. The pixels are assigned lifetimes at random from a first order Erlang distribution:

$$e(t) = \lambda \cdot e^{-\lambda \cdot t} \qquad (2)$$

e(t) is the probability for a pixel to degrade at time, t, while λ is a degradation rate constant. Once its lifetime has expired, a pixel is considered degraded. From equation 2 lifetimes are picked at random according to a Monte Carlo algorithm (Göpferich and Langer, 1993). The difference between surface eroding and bulk eroding polymers is taken into account with a condition that

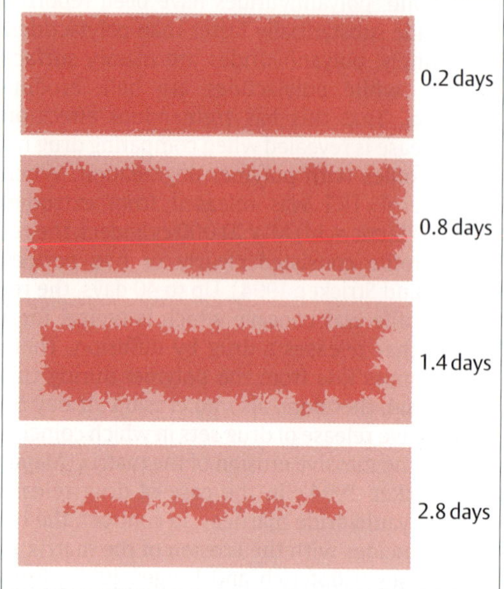

Fig. 3 Simulation of the erosion of a surface-eroding polymer cross-section. Reproduced with permission from (Göpferich and Langer, 1995).

must be fulfilled prior to calculating lifetimes. While for a surface eroding polymer pixel the lifetime is calculated only after contact with the erosion medium, for a bulk eroding polymer lifetimes are calculated right from the beginning of the experiment. Then pixels are degraded in the sequence of their lifetimes. The difference between surface erosion and bulk erosion is again of importance when pixels are eroded. In the case of a surface eroding polymer, degraded pixels can erode immediately. For a bulk eroding polymer, degraded pixels can only erode after they establish contact to a pore. Figure **3** shows an example for the simulation of the erosion of a matrix that consists of surface eroding polymer only. Such simulations have been used to describe the erosion of polyanhydrides (Göpferich and Langer, 1993).

Although it seems that such models could be applied only to the investigation of erosion phenomena, they can also be used for the simulation of erosion-controlled drug release. One simply assumes that whenever a pixel erodes a relative amount of 1/gridsize is released. This is sufficiently accurate if diffusion and other processes are so fast that they have no impact on the release kinetics. Making this simple assumption it was possible to show that the model is able to predict drug release from polyanhydrides such as poly(1,3-bis[*p*-carboxyphenoxy]propane-co-sebacic acid) (Göpferich and Langer, 1995). This good agreement between erosion (model) and drug release (experiment) illustrates that the assumption regarding release is valid for fast eroding polymers in combination with hydrophilic low molecular weight drugs. If other phenomena affect drug release in addition to erosion, diffusion theory has to be used to describe the release of drugs.

Erosion-Controlled Drug Release from Degradable Polymers

There are numerous examples for the development of controlled release dosage forms made of biodegradable polymers in the contemporary literature. Trying to give a detailed survey on all these systems is almost impossible. It is rather the intention of this chapter to illustrate with an example the way that surface and bulk eroding polymers function. Taking advantage of the properties of surface eroding polymers such as polyanhydrides attempts were made to release substances in a preprogrammed way. Such drug release behavior is interesting for a number of therapies such as local tumor therapy or vaccination. The advantages for the first application are the prevention of tumor cell resistance against continuously administered cytostatics and the application of drugs at the right time for biopharmaceutic reasons. To prevent the development of tolerance during the application of an implant one can, for example, release two drugs one after another. An example that illustrates the need for releasing a drug out of an implant at the right time is the therapy of brain tumors. Investigations on the distribution of drugs after the implantation of drug-loaded biodegradable polymer matrices at the tumor site revealed that most of the released drug is cleared from the tumor site rapidly by convection (Kalyanasundaram, 1996). After a couple of days convection slows down and increases the availability of drug again. Therefore, the release patterns where a dose of drug is released initially and another after convection has slowed down would be beneficial. The same release profile has a tremendous potential for the purpose of vaccination.

Both release patterns could theoretically be obtained from matrices made of surface eroding polymers. When such matrices consists of two polymer layers one should first have the release of drug from the mantle and then out of the core. If both layers are loaded with different drugs it should be possible to achieve their release one after another. Although it is possible to manufacture such matrices (Göpferich et al., 1995), they would have large dimensions when one would intend to postpone the release of the second dose for more than a couple of days. It is, therefore, rather desirable to postpone the release of the second dose by another mechanism than surface erosion alone (Göpferich, 1997). This means in return that a slow eroding polymer has to be used to separate the two drug-loaded surface-eroding polymer layers. Such polymers are usually bulk eroding. An example for a composite polymer matrix is shown in Figure **4a**. A bulk eroding layer of poly(D,L-lactic acid) is used

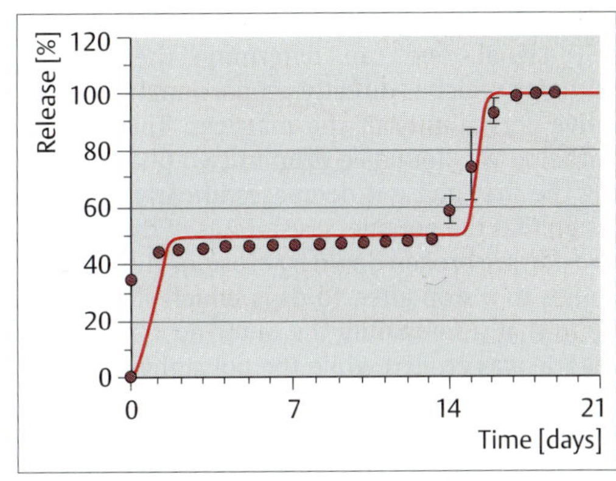

Fig. **5** Fit of the erosion model (line) to the experimental data for drug release (filled circles) from composite matrices. Reproduced with permission from (Göpferich, 1997).

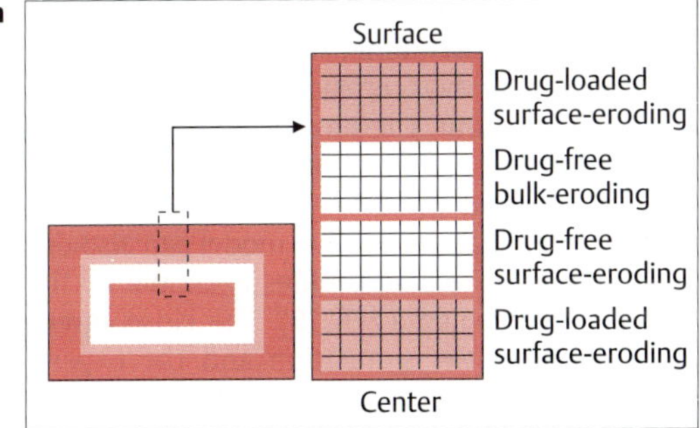

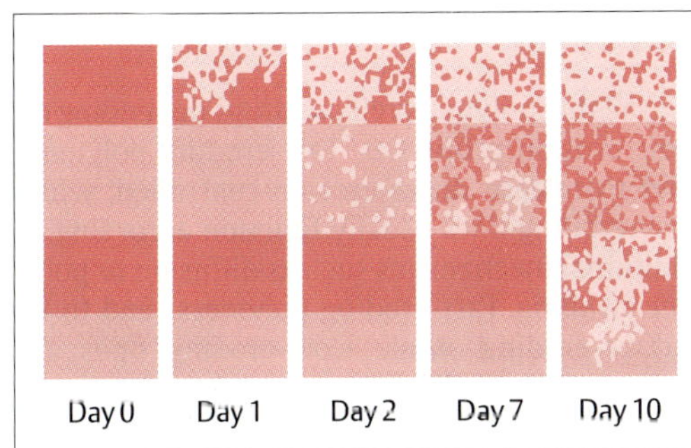

Fig. **4** **(a)** Structure of a composite polymer matrix disc and its representation by two-dimensional grid. Reproduced with permission from (Göpferich, 1997). **(b)** Erosion time-series for a composite polyanhydride matrix disc. Non-eroded polymer is shown in black and gray to distinguish the various layers of the matrix, pores are shown in white and pores inside the bulk-eroding polymer layer that are connected to the surface are shown in black. Reproduced with permission from (Göpferich, 1997).

there to slow down erosion on its way into the core of the matrix that carries the second dose. An example for a drug release profile is shown in Figure **5**. The release of a model compound (brilliant blue) is clearly proceeding in two phases. During an initial phase of 2 days, half of the total dose is released while the second half is released after a 12-day period of no release. If the dose inside the core were replaced by another drug, it is obvious that a release profile would be obtained where the drugs are released one after another.

Although the system works quite well it is essential to understand how the release is controlled. The release of drug during the first phase is probably erosion-controlled as the released dye stems from the surface eroding polymer mantle. The release of the second dose is, however, not readily understandable. It is, for example, possible that not only erosion is controlling the second period of drug release but also osmotic effects. The poly(D,L-lactic acid) layer could, for example, behave as a semi-permeable membrane that lets water pass into the core but that does not allow the release of degradation products from inside. This would lead to a constantly increasing osmotic pressure and the rupture of the membrane followed by the spontaneous release of the second dose of drug. As an alternative to this mechanism, drug release could be controlled by the erosion of the anhydride layers while the delay of the second release period could be controlled by the slow erosion of the polylactide layer. To verify one of the two hypothesis, the erosion of drug-free composite matrices was investigated by differential scanning calorimetry (DSC). From the DSC signal, one can determine the melting enthalpy which is directly proportional to the relative crystallinity of the matrices. The melting enthalpy was found to drop in two phases. During the first phase it decreases linearly which is a sign that the polymer crystallites of the polyanhydride are broken down by erosion. This process comes to a stop after 10 days which shows that up to that time mainly the outermost anhydride mantle was eroded while the polyanhydride layers inside are still intact. As the release of drugs from within the implant has not yet started at this point, one can conclude that the PLA layer is still in place. Between days 10 and 14, the crystallinity increases again. This is not because new crystalline polymer is created, but because the degradation products of the mantle leave during this period and decrease the amount of amorphous material. In return one can conclude that the crystallinity that is attributed to the core of the matrix is not affected by erosion, which means that the poly(D,L-lactic acid) layer is still protecting the core. The secondary maximum of crystallinity coincides with the onset of drug release from the implant. This suggests that the release of the second dose proceeds also erosion-controlled. From these studies one can conclude that the overall kinetics of drug release are mainly controlled by erosion.

Modeling the erosion of this composite device supported this hypothesis. For the composite matrices, a model was developed that accounts for the erosion of bulk-eroding polymers as well. For modeling the erosion of composite polymer matrices, their cross-sections were first represented theoretically by a two-dimensional rectangular grid as schematically shown in Fig. **4a.** It covers only half of the matrix in the vertical direction because the erosion problem is symmetric with respect to the axes of the cylinder. To reduce the amount of necessary calculations further, the grid covers only a part of the matrix in the horizontal direction which is sufficiently accurate for large discs. For the development of an erosion algorithm, it had to be distinguished between surface-eroding polymer layers and bulk-eroding ones because they show different erosion behavior. For pixels located inside a surface-eroding polyanhydride layer the erosion-condition was again that contact to the degradation medium was established. Lifetimes were again sampled from first order Erlang distributions. To simulate the erosion of bulk-eroding polymer this

algorithm had to be modified. It was assumed that all pixels in this layer have equal opportunity to erode after at least one pixel representing bulk-eroding polymer has contact to the erosion medium. Finally, all pixels were removed from the grid in the sequence of their lifetimes. The result of a simulation is shown in Figure **4b.** For reasons of simplicity only a limited number of pixels was used. Erosion starts on the surface of the implant but does not affect the bulk-eroding polymer layer until it comes into contact with a pore. After 1 day this contact is established and after 2 days the bulk-eroding polymer layer has visibly eroded. The surface-eroding polyanhydride layer underneath is not affected by erosion at that time because there is no immediate contact to the erosion medium. After 7 days, when a percolation cluster stretches through the bulk-eroding polymer, erosion spreads into the core of the implant. For the formation of such a connecting pore, approximately half of the pixels must be eroded on a two-dimensional grid (Stauffer, 1985). After 10 days, erosion proceeds into core of the implant. The simulation suggests that the polylactide layer functions as a time fuse that is responsible for the delay of the release of the second dose. That the erosion model can also describe the drug release profiles is shown by fitting it to release data (Fig. **5**). The close agreement between the simulation and the experimental data supports the experimental finding that the device is mainly erosion-controlled.

Conclusions

Degradable polymers release drugs depending on their erosion properties. Fast-eroding polymers tend to release drugs erosion-controlled, while slow-eroding ones usually function according to additional mechanisms such as diffusion or polymer swelling. Fast-eroding polymers tend to be surface-eroding, while slow-eroding ones are bulk-eroding. Both properties are useful in the area of drugs release which was illustrated with an example for the programmable release of drugs from implants. Surface erosion as well as bulk erosion can be modeled using mathematical models. Such models allow one to describe erosion as well as erosion-controlled drug release even for polymer matrices that are made of both polymer types.

Acknowledgements

Thanks are due to the Deutsche Forschungsgemeinschaft (DGF) who supported parts of this project with research grant GO 565/3 – 1 and to Scios Nova and Boehringer Ingelheim for providing the polymers.

References

Albertsson AC: The shape of the biodegradation curve for low and high density polyethenes in prolonged series of experiments. Europ Pol J 1980; 16: 623 – 30.

Brunner A, Göpferich A. Problems concerning peptide stability in PLA/GA microspheres, CRS Conference on Advances in Controlled Delivery, Baltimore, U.S.A., Conference Proceedings 1996: 39 – 40.

Göpferich A, Langer R. Modeling of polymer erosion in three dimensions – rotationally symmetric devices, AIChE Journal 1995; 41: 2292 – 9.

Göpferich A, Langer R. Polymer erosion. Macromolecules 1993; 26: 4105 – 12.

Göpferich A. Mechanism of polymer degradation and elimination. In: Domb A, Kost J, Wiseman D. (eds.). Handbook of Biodegradable Polymers. Harwood Acad. Publ. Inc., in press 1996 b.

Göpferich A. Polymer degradation and erosion: mechanisms and applications. Eur J Pharm Biopharm 1996; 42: 1 – 11.

Göpferich A, Shieh L, Langer R. Aspects of polymer erosion. Mat Res Soc Symp Proc 1995; 394: 155 – 60.

Göpfert A. The erosion of composite polymer matrices. Biomaterials, in press 1997.

Kalyanasundaram S, Zhao Z, Sills A, Brem H, Leong KW. Controlled release for immunotherapy: analysis of intracranial transport of IL-2. 23 rd Intern. Symp Control Rel Bioact Mater, Kyoto, Japan 1996; 23: 230 – 1.

Langer R. New methods of drug delivery. Science 1990; 249: 1527 – 32.

Langer R, Vacanti J. Tissue engineering. Science 1993; 260: 920 – 6.

Leenslang J, Pennings A, Ruud R, Rozema F, Boering G. Resorbable materials of poly(L-lactide). VI. Plates and screws for internal fracture fixation. Biomaterials 1987; 8: 70 – 3.

Mayer U, Stricker H. Wirkstoffhaltige Träger aus poly-D,L-lactiden. Krankenhauspharmazie 1994; 15: 596 – 600.

Stauffer D. Introduction to percolation theory, Taylor & Francis, London 1985.

Tamada J, Langer R. Erosion mechanism of hydrolytically degradable polymers. Proc Nat Acad Sci 1993; 90: 552 – 6.

Zygourakis K. Discrete simulations and bioerodible controlled release systems. Polym Prepr (Am Chem Soc, Div. Polym Chem) 1989; 30: 456 – 7.

First Results with a New Class of Bioresorbable Oligomers and Visions

H.-J. Pfefferle

Introduction

In this chapter a new class of bioresorbable material is described. Some examples of our research show that this new class of oligomers is characterized by interesting properties and possibilities of application.

Concerning the working field of resorbable polymers, Merck Biomaterial concentrates on three principle aims:

- Occlusion material for bleeding bone wounds,
- Drug delivery systems, and
- Bone glue.

The starting point of our considerations, was the well-known and extensively investigated polylactic acid. Polylactic acid (Fig. 1 a) is a linear polyester, consisting of lactic acid monomer units. It can be adjusted to a molecular weight range, which is as wide as 2,000 up to 1 million g/mole. Some preparations based on these polymers, are approved for the parenteral application in humans. For example, resorbable bone-screws or slow-releasing hormone preparations contain polylactic acid.

The Material

However, the polylactic acid did not serve our purpose. So we came to this new class of oligomers (Fig. 1 b). These oligomers are composed of two components. On the one hand a multi-functional alcohol like ethyleneglycol or glycerine, on the other hand, lactic or glycolic acid. However, for the synthesis, we use the cyclic dimers and not the free acids, because of a more favorable reaction course. All following specifications, which refer to the molecular ratio of composition, are related to these acid-dimers. So a glycero-oligolactide 1 : 18 has 36 molecules lactic acid per one molecule glycerine.

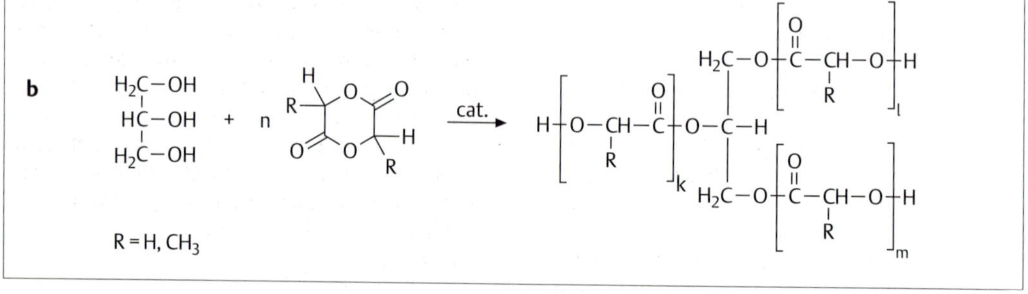

Fig. 1 Structures of the new oligomers.

The alcohol in the oligomer acts on the one hand as a branching-point for the molecular chain, on the other hand as an internal plastifier. So we obtain a branched oligomer, which ranges in molecular weight from 300 up to 6000 g/mole.

Both the low molecular weight and the branched structure, lead to a lower viscosity and a lower glass transition temperature, compared to similar polymers.

One of the advantages of these oligomers is the possibility to adjust the molecular weight within quite exact margins by choosing an appropriate mixture of starting materials. This is a fundamental method to control consistency and degradation-rate. Later on you will see that there are still other possibilities to influence material properties. In Table **1** the range of consistency, which it is possible to choose is given. The range begins at the lower end with the viscosity of maple syrup. The upper end of the range is marked by a material which is as brittle as glass at room temperature. But, when warmed with the fingers, it can be moulded like beeswax.

Table **1**   Consistency of the oligomers

moles lactide per 1 mole glycerine	consistency at 20 °C like	typical mol. mass
0.5	maple syrup	300
2	acacia honey	700
5	beeswax	1 000
18	glass; at 37 °C like beeswax	5 900

The degradation rates of the oligomers correlate with their molecular weight, however, the crystalline properties and the shape of the surface also have a great influence. Two examples should show the extreme points of possible degradation profiles we can adjust by varying molecular mass and copolymers.

A glycero-oligo-lactide/glycolide with 4 molecules L-lactic acid and 2 molecules glycolic acid per 1 molecule glycerine (GOLG 1:2:1) has a molecule mass of about 700 g/mole. It degrades within two days to the amount of 90 % and after further 12 days it has completely disappeared. The degradation was followed by determination of lactic and glycolic acid in the release-medium by HPLC.

Another oligomer, the GOL 1:18, with a molecular mass of about 5900 g/mole has a considerably longer degradation time. After 120 days just 50 % has degraded.

Within these margins it is possible to adjust the degradation time by varying the compounds of the oligomer. Moreover, it is possible to modify the properties by blending the oligomers with different additives. Our development of an occlusion material for bleeding bone wounds is a good example for this.

Applications

Bleeding Bone Wounds

We looked for a material with the following properties:
- Well-tolerated by tissue,
- Sufficiently effective (in stopping bleedings),
- Easy to administer,
- Fast degradation.

One of the problems we encountered here was the marked stickiness of the pure polymer to medical gloves. So we systematically blended the oligomer with some additives like:
- Hydroxyapatite,
- Calcium carbonate,
- Polyethyleneglycol,
- Phospholipone H 100,
- Cetyl palmitate.

We came to a mixture of a low-molecular-weight oligomer, with a well-tolerated additive. This material does not adhere to gloves and further it met all our requirements, including the possibility of simple manufacturing.

Drug Delivery Systems

The interesting properties of these oligomers also open new possibilities in drug delivery systems. Such a system releases a drug over a certain time range after implantation. The drug-release depends on degradation of polymer, drug-diffusion in the polymer, or both factors.

There are a few possibilities for loading a polymer with drugs and to bring it in form which is applicable. The most important procedures for manufacturing loaded polymers are:
- Melting,
- Compressing,
- Extruding, and
- Dissolving.

The melting of polymers with drugs has a small consumption of material and the molten mass can be prepared in few different forms. But one has to regard the thermal stress for polymer and drug. In the case of our oligomers the thermal stress is a minor problem because the low softening-temperature allows us to incorporate drugs at a comparatively low temperature.

By compressing a mixture of pulverized polymer with drug in a tablet-press we obtain an implantable polymer-tablet. Depending on pressure the tablet acquires a differently porous surface which controls the drug-release in the first place.

The extrusion, a kind of injection moulding, offers a great variety of different shapes, like little rods, tapes or tubes, and the possibility to produce in a large-scale. A mixture of a polymer-solution with a solution or a suspension of the drug in the same solvent, can be formed in different moulds. After removing the solvent we receive a form which contains varying amounts of the constituents. Thus, each of these methods has its pros and cons and influences to a certain extent the material properties and drug release.

It is also possible to give the oligomers a consistency of an ointment. This offers new possibilities in the application of drugs. Hence, it is possible to spread such a bioresorbable ointment onto an operation field, or it can simply be injected.

Results

The next three diagrams show examples of *in-vitro* drug-release profiles. They differ in oligomer composition, shape of system, and drug substance. Figure **2** shows the release of gentamicin from melted pin. After 9 days, 90% of the drug was delivered. The melting process leads to a smooth surface of the pin, and the start of release is delayed, until after an initial swelling-phase.

The release of methotrexate from a pasty system (Fig. **3**) is mainly controlled by drug diffusion. This can be observed on account of the orange color of the methotrexate, which clearly marks the diffusion layer. Up to the fortieth, day, sixty percent of the drug was delivered.

The release of a cyclic peptide from a pressed tablet (Fig. **4**) is marked by an initial burst of drug substance, within the first hours. This is because the drug particles are sited on the surface, not covered by oligomer.

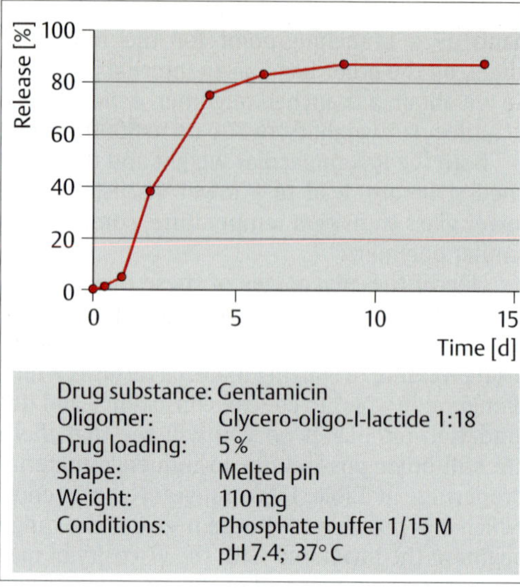

Drug substance: Gentamicin
Oligomer: Glycero-oligo-l-lactide 1:18
Drug loading: 5 %
Shape: Melted pin
Weight: 110 mg
Conditions: Phosphate buffer 1/15 M
                pH 7.4; 37° C

Fig. **2**   Gentamicin release from a melted pin.

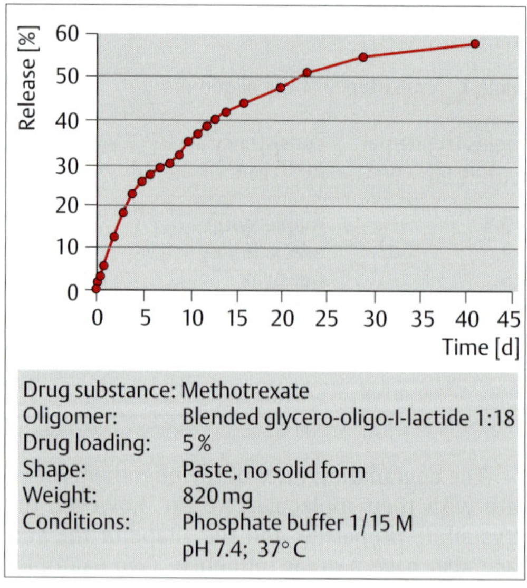

Drug substance: Methotrexate
Oligomer: Blended glycero-oligo-l-lactide 1:18
Drug loading: 5 %
Shape: Paste, no solid form
Weight: 820 mg
Conditions: Phosphate buffer 1/15 M
                pH 7.4; 37° C

Fig. **3**   Release of methotrexate from a paste.

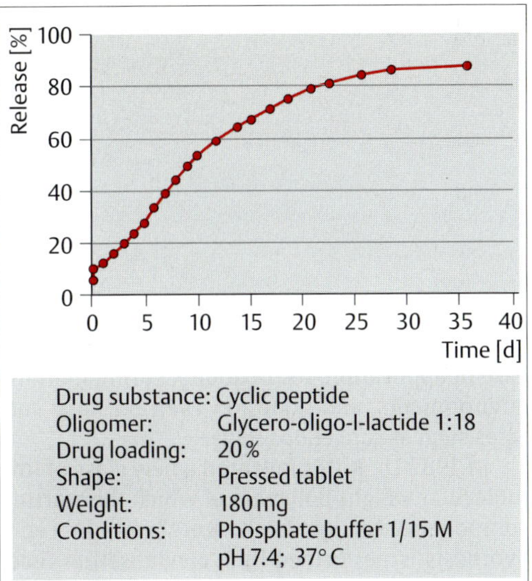

Fig. **4**   Relese of a cyclic peptide from a pressed tablet.

Visions

It follows from this that, in addition to the high solid polymers, also the soft oligomers can also be employed in surgical interventions. Finally, the possible applications of this new class of oligomers are summarized:

- Use as an occlusion material for bleeding bone wounds;
- Use as drug delivery system with new properties;
- Coating of other materials;
- Use as an additive to modify other materials;
- Basic material uses for reactive polymers like a bone glue.

Conclusions

The outstanding features of these oligomers are summarized here:

- Favorable properties for manufacturing, handling, and application,
- The possibility to adjust the drug delivery and the degradation rate in broad ranges.

First Results with a Bioresorbable Bone Glue

R. Wenz

Introduction

Glueing is an attractive technique to link divided materials as it is easy and rapid to perform instead of using nails, screws and pins to connect fractured bone. The advantages of using a glue are an optimal load transfer from one fracture side to the other because a connection is made over the whole surface and not only a spotted contact as when using pins.

Moreover, in cases of fractures involving joints where an uneveness of the articular surface may arise, this uneveness can be compensated through the adhesive seam. Another potential advantage is the avoidance of stress-protection in fracture repair by using an elastic glue instead of metallic implants with high rigidity and stiffness.

A favorable effect upon fracture-healing could also be the undisturbed blood supply, especially from the periosteal side in contrast to metal osteosynthesis.

Bioresorbable Bone Glues

The first attempts to develop a bone-glueing system come from Egypt and are more than 4000 years old. Centuries later in 1772, plaster of Paris was introduced, which is still used today for fracture fixation. Other developments were epoxide-resins, cyanoacrylates, polyurethanes, and the fibrin glues. These premature developments failed because they did not meet medical requirements such as biocompatibility, stability during storage, lack of systemic and local toxicity, sterilizable, ease of application, resorbability, curing in moist environments, and adhesion even on fatty surfaces such as cancellous bone.

In 1982 Dr. Ritter invented a new class of low molecular weight polymers of which the starting components for synthesis are shown in Fig. 1. Synthesis is performed by a condensation reaction of a multifunctional alcohol, for example the bifunctional alcohol ethyleneglycol shown in Figure **1**, and oligomers of lactic acid, generated by an acidic ring opening reaction of lactide, the dimer of lactic acid. In a second reaction, this non-reactive condensation product, ethyleneglycol-oligolactide, is esterified with methacrylic acid, thus producing a highly reactive end-product with methacrylic end groups, which is stabilized by α-tocopherol (Fig. **2**).

The highly viscous macromolecule can be easily polymerized through irradiation either with a photoinitiator and irradiation with high-energy light, chemically, or by ionizing radiation (Fig. **3**). Figure **3** represents only one side of the polymerized molecule of Figure **2** for the sake of a simplified image of the molecules in polymerization.

Since in surgery an easy handling is desirable, a system had to be developed which allows an *in situ* curing without additional aids like irradiation. Therefore, we used in our development a two-component system, one component representing the glue in the unpolymerized, but highly viscous form and, as the second component, the non-reactive oligomer without reactive end

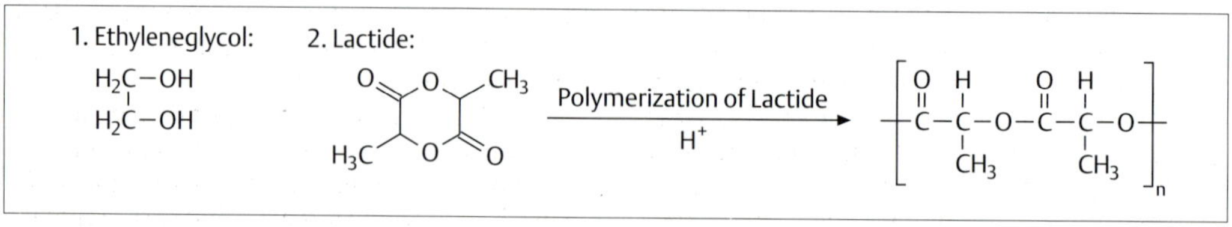

Fig. **1** Synthesis of bone glue.

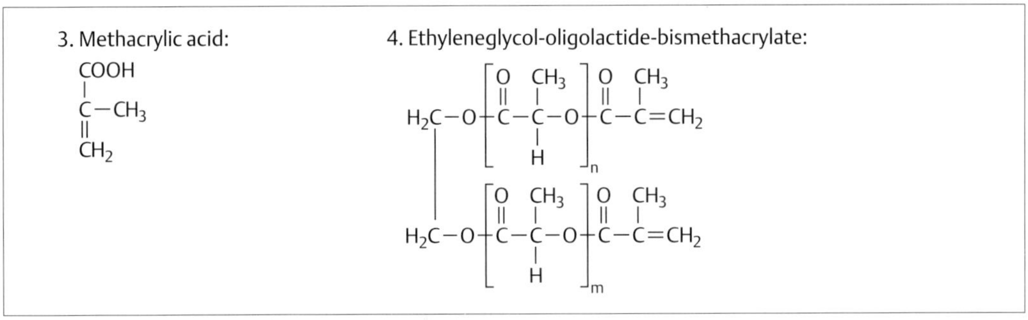

3. Methacrylic acid:

COOH
|
C—CH₃
‖
CH₂

4. Ethyleneglycol-oligolactide-bismethacrylate:

Fig. **2**   Synthesis of bone glue with methacrylic acid.

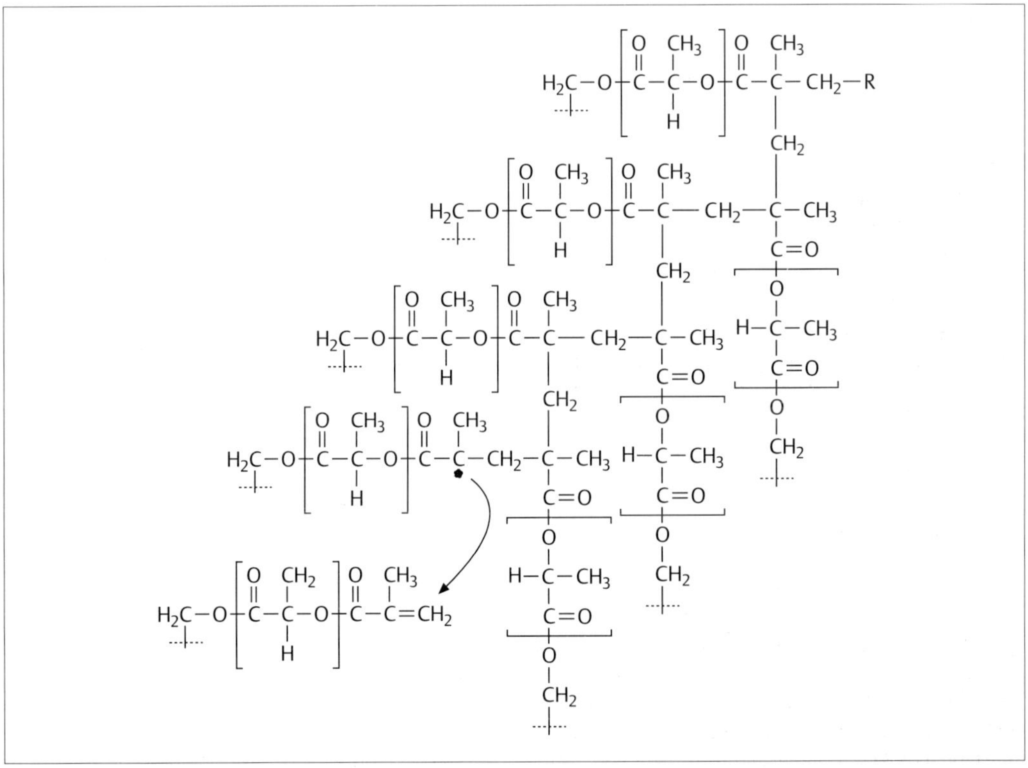

Fig. **3**   Bone glue polymerization process.

groups. This second component contains a solubilized alkyl boron, which acts as a radical donor, thus initiating the polymerization process.

Since the solidified glue is decomposed via hydrolysis of the ester bonds, a not-cell driven process, the term bioresorbability applies mainly to the degradation products. Figure **4** demonstrates the degradation products which result after hydrolytic cleavage. Ethyleneglycol as well

as lactic acid are well known metabolites of the mammallian metabolism where they enter the Krebs-Henseleit-cycle to be excreted entirely as carbon dioxide and water.

The larger molecule of Figure **4,** of which only half of the molecule is represented, is an oligomer/polymer of methacylic acid, remaining after hydrolysis. Such oligomers, which are highly water-soluble, can be excreted via the kidneys, pro-

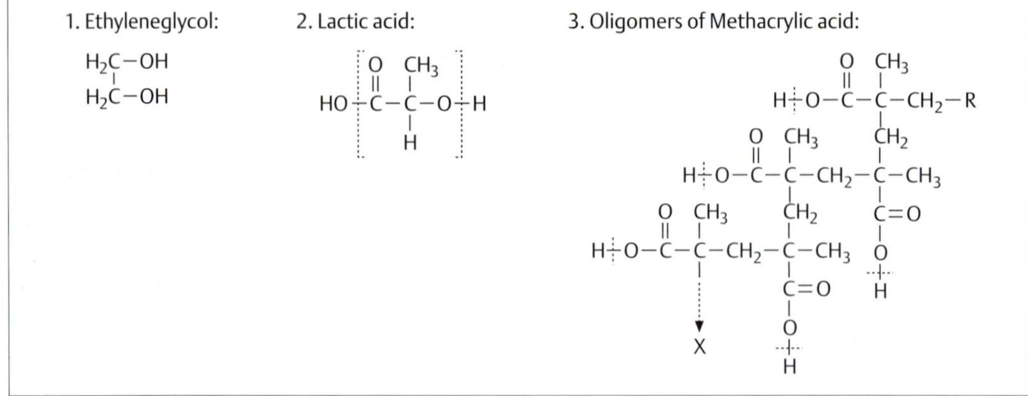

Fig. **4** End products of hydrolytic cleavage.

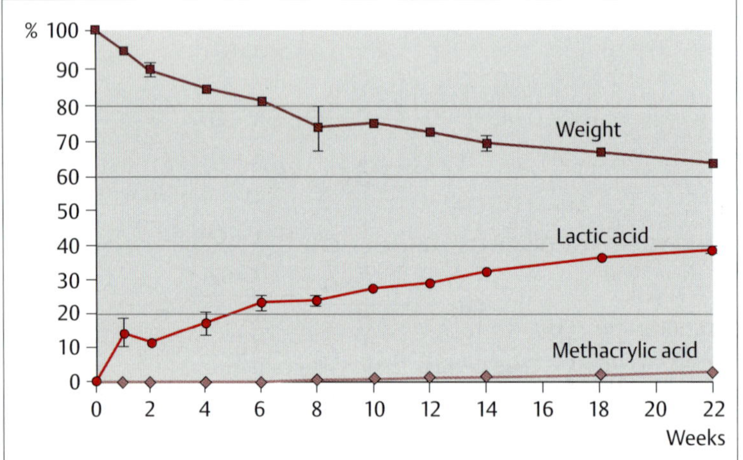

Fig. **5** Weight loss in phosphate-buffered saline.

vided that their molecular weight is less than approximately 8000.

For these methacylate oligomers it seems certain that they do not reach such high molecular weights, due to steric inhibition during the polymerization process (Fig. **3**).

Because of this steric inhibition an entanglement of differently elongated ethyleneglycol-oligolactide-bismethacrylate oligomers and polymers, respectively, is achieved. Therefore, the degradation behavior is quite different in comparison to high-molecular-weight polymers like poly-L-lactide and is strongly dependent on the polymerization procedure applied in the preparation.

For example, with a γ-polymerized glue we recorded a weight loss of about 40% within 22 weeks in phosphate-buffered saline (pH 7.4). The decrease in weight was almost linear. If polymerization is induced chemically, for example, by boron-alkylates, we found a weight loss of 40% within 70 days (Fig. **5**). The decrease in weight is in good correlation with the increase of lactic acid, as the main component of the molecule (expressed in percentage of initial weight), in the storage buffer.

The reasons for the stickiness of a glue are characterized through adhesion properties, which are of physical, chemical, unspecific mechanical origin, and the cohesion force, which is an inherent property of the glue. The cohesion is directly dependent on the chemical and physical bonds between the polymer chains which, in turn, are dependent on the viscosity of the unpo-

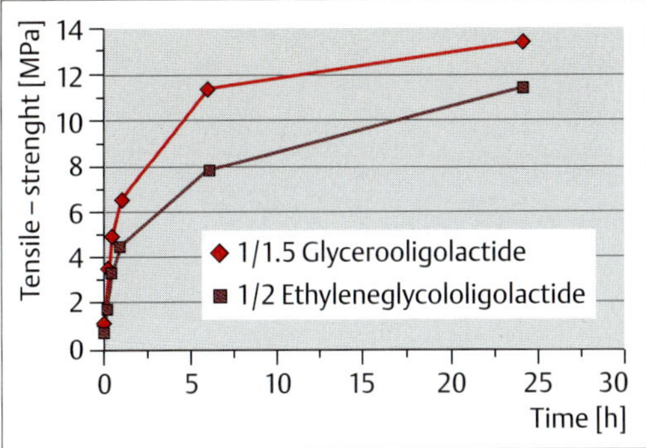

Fig. **6** Tensile strengths.

lymerized macromolecule through influence on the dimensions of the polymer chains generated during polymerization. This is demonstrated in Figure **6**. The macromolecule, ethyleneglycol-oligolactide-bismethacrylate, which has much lower viscosity than its counterpart with the higher alcohol glycerol, yields a better cohesion, expressed as tensile strength. As polymerization acts as an exothermic reaction, we do not reach polymerization temperatures more than 40 °C, and therefore we do not generate a necrotic interface between bone and glue.

The indications to use such a medical glue are fractures contributed to joints together with a joint bridging fixation, fractures with only little soft-tissue coverage, applications in the field of oral-facial surgery, and in parodontology.

Conclusions

Since the polymer glue is a biocompatible and resorbable material, it is possible to incorporate bioactive drugs and use the glue for a drug delivery system. For the present we tested the release properties of the glue for the antibiotic gentamicin and for the cytostatic drug methotrexate. In both cases we achieved a good release kinetics with an almost linear increase of the drug in the elution buffer due to the degradation behavior of the polymeric glue in aqueous solutions. Therefore this *in situ* curing, moldable material may be of use as a therapeutic system, for therapy of osteomyelitis and soft-tissue infections, or as a carrier matrix for the low-dose therapy of osteoarthritis.

Index